CAUTION AGAINST CANCER

DR. RAVINDRA KUMAR

RIGI PUBLICATION

CAUTION AGAINST CANCER

BY

DR. RAVINDRA KUMAR

Originally Published in India

ISBN: 978-93-89540-97-0

Published by RIGI PUBLICATION

PRINTER: RIGI PRINTERS

777, Street no.9, Krishna Nagar
Khanna-141401 (Punjab), India
Website: www.rigipublication.com
Email: info@rigipublication.com
Phone: +91-9357710014, +91-9465468291

FOREWORD

Cancer is a word that carries a weight and a fear that few others can match. It is a journey that millions of individuals and their loved ones embark upon each year, a journey marked by uncertainty, courage, and resilience.

It is gratifying to note that Dr. Ravinder Kumar has delved into this complicated issue of cancer. He has written an excellent and authentic book on cancer.

The book has a total of 20 chapters. The opening chapter is devoted to history of Cancer. He has covered almost all types of cancers in quite detail. In these pages, author has explored the multifaceted aspects of cancer, its biology, its impact on individuals and families, and prevention, and perhaps most importantly, the resilience of the human spirit when faced with this formidable adversary. Author has done well to bring relevant knowledge about the cancer for the masses. Challenges on the cancer front are many and even complicated ones.

The book will be useful for a patient seeking knowledge, a caregiver in need of guidance, or simply someone curious about this complex disease, I hope this book serves as a source of information, inspiration, and, above all, a reminder that even in the darkest of times, there is always a glimmer of hope.

I am sure like his many other books by the author for the general masses, this book will also be very useful for better awareness of cancer.

Prof. M U Rabbhani

Former Dean, Faculty of Medicine

Jawaharlal Nehru Medical College

A.M.U. Aligarh

AUTHOR'S DESK

- I wish to share my knowledge among the masses on cancer awareness through this book titled "Caution Against Cancer". Because cancer is a dreaded disease and it's symptoms mimics other diseases, it is hard to diagnose. Hopefully with the help of this book people can early detect the disease and have higher survival rate.

- Opening of this of the book is devoted to history of cancer as it shows different theories in connection with cancer and how it came into existence.

- Cancer is the most common cause of the death in the United States of America.

- There are five broad categories of indicate the tissue and blood classification:

i. **Carcinoma:** Carcinoma accounts for 80 to 90 percent of all cancer cases such as Melanoma, Basal Cell carcinoma, squamous cell skin cancer.

ii. Sarcoma: Types of sarcoma include:
Soft tissue, Osteosarcoma, Ewing's sarcoma and Chondrosarcomas.

iii. **lymphoma:** Types of lymphoma include: Hodgkin's lymphoma and Cutaneous lymphoma.

iv. Leukemia and their types.

v. **Myeloma:** Myeloma cells collect in many bones forming many tumours. This is called multiple myeloma.

- The reason for writing the book was that my wife Upasana suffered a lot and this dreaded disease took her life. My children Manasi and Mahima took very keen interest to help me write this book. I can't forget my colleague Prof. MU Rabbani for Dean Faculty of Medicine Jawahar Lal Nehru Medical College, AMU, Aligarh, who also provided me lot of help for writing this book. Dr Satish Kumar, having more than 40 years of experience in the field of Medical Science, also inspired me to write such a book.

Dr. Ravindra Kumar former Scientist, CSIR.

CAUTION AGAINST CANCER

INDEX

CHAPTER 1

HISTORY OF CANCER

The disease was first called by Greek Physician Hippocrates (460-370 BC). He is considered the " Father of Medicine" Hippocrates used the terms Carcinos and Carcinoma to describe non-ulcer-forming tumors. In Greek this means a Crab.

Hippocrates is credited with naming "Cancer" as "Karkinoma" (Carcinoma) because a Tumor looked like a 'Crab'

Types of cancer are named for organs or tissues where the cancer form. For example, lung cancer starts in the lung, and brain cancer starts in the brain. Cancer also may be described by the type of cell that formed them, such as an epithelial cell.

Latin cancer is the generic word for 'Crab'. According to the Greek myth is based on the Karkinos (Greek "Cancer"), a Crab crushed under the foot of the Heracles, and whose remains were placed in the sky by Hera, forming the cancer constellation.

Some of the earliest evidence of cancer is found among fossilized bone tumors, human mummies in ancient Egypt, and ancient manuscripts. Growths and suggestive of the bone cancer called Osteosarcoma have been seen in mummies. Bony skull destruction as seen in the cancer of the head and neck has been found, too.

British library, and several other sources of information on the cancer in Indian history.

Paleopathology studies from Indus Valley civilization sites do not reveal any malignancy.

Cancer like diseases and remedies are mentioned in ancient Ayurveda and Siddha manuscripts from India.

Cancer was rarely mentioned in medieval literature from India. Cancer case reports from India began in the 17th century. Between 1860 and 1910, several audits and cancer case series were published by Indian Medical Doctors across India.

Landmark study by Nath and Grewal used autopsy, pathology, and clinical data between 1917 and 1932 from various Medical College and hospitals across India to confirm that cancer was a common cause of death in the middle aged and elderly Indians. India's cancer burden has apparently low as a result of the short life expectancy of the natives in those times. In 1946, a national committee on health reforms recommended the creation of sufficient facilities to diagnose and manage the increasing the cancer burden in all Indian states Trends from the Mumbai population-based cancer registry revealed a four - fold increase in the patients with cancer from 1964 to 2012.

Depending on the epidemiologic transition level, wide interstate variation in cancer burden is found in India.

Cancer has been recognised in India since antiquity. India's current burden of million incident cancers in the result of an epidemiologic transition, improved cancer diagnostics, and improved cancer data capture. The increase in the cancer in India with wide interstate variations offers useful insights and important lessons for developing countries in managing their increasing cancer burdens.

The study of cancer, called oncology, is the work of countless doctors and scientists around the world whose discoveries in anatomy, physiology, chemistry, epidemiology, and other related fields made oncology what it is today. Technological advances and the ever-increasing understanding of cancer make this field one of the most rapidly involving areas of modern medicine.

Growth in our knowledge of the cancer biology has led to remarkable progress in cancer prevention, early detection, and treatment. Scientists have learned in the centuries preceding. This doesn't change the fact, however, that all scientific knowledge is based on the knowledge already acquired by hard work the discovery of our predecessor and we know that there is still a lot more to learn.

Understanding cancer causes: Ancient time to present

Theories about cancer causes.

Early theories about cancer causes: From the ancient times, physicians have puzzled over the causes of cancer. Ancient Egyptians blamed cancers on the Gods.

Humoral theory:

Hippocrates believed that the body had 4 humours (body fluids): blood, phlegm, yellow bile, and black bile. When the humans were balanced, a person was healthy. The belief was that too much or too little of any of the humours caused disease. An excess of the black bile in various body sites was thought to cause cancer. This theory of the cancer was passed on by the Romans and was enhanced by the influential doctor Galen's medical teaching, which remained the unchallenged standard through the middle ages for over 1300 years.

During the period, the study of the body, including autopsies, was prohibited for religious reasons, which limited progress of medical knowledge.

Lymph theory: Among theories that replaced humoral theories of cancer was the formation of cancer by another body fluid, lymph. Life was believed to consist of continuous and appreciate movement of the fluid parts of the body through the solid parts of all the fluids, the most important were blood and lymph. Stahi and Hoffman theorized that cancer was composed of fermenting and degerating lymph, varying in density, acidity, and alkalinity. The lymph theory gained rapid support, John Hunter, the Scottish surgeon from the 1700s, agreed that tumors grow from lymph constantly thrown out by the blood.

Blastema theory: In 1838, German pathologist Johannes Muller demonstrated that cancer is made up of cells and and not lymph, but he believed that cancer cell did not come from normal cells. Muller proposed that cancer cell devloped form budding elements (Blastema) between normal tissues. His student, Rudolph Virchow (1821-1902), the famous General pathologist, determined that all cells, including cancer cells, are derived from other cells.

Chronic irritation theory: Virchow proposed that chronic irritation was the cause of cancer, but he believed incorrectly that cancers " spread like a liqui". In the 1860 s German surgeon, Karl Thiersch, showed that cancer metastasize cells and not through the spread of malignant cells not through the some unidentified fluid.

Trauma theory:

Despite advances in the understanding of cancer, from the late 1800s untill the 1920, Trauma was thought by some of the cause cancer.

This belief was maintained despite of failure of injury to cause cancer in experimental animals.

Infectious theory:

Zacutus Lusitani (1575-1674) and Nicholas Tulp (1593-1674), two Doctors in Holland, concluded at almost the same time that cancer was contagious. They made this conclusion based on their experiences with a breast Cancer in members of the some house hold.

Lusitani and Tulp publicized the contagious theory in 1649 and 1652, respectively. They proposed that cancer patients should be isolated, preferably outside the cities and towns, in order to prevent the spread of cancer.

Throughout the 17th and 18th centuries, some believed that cancer was contagious. In fact, the first cancer hospital in France was forced to move from the city in 1779 because people feared cancer would spread throughout the city. Although human cancer, itself is not contagious.

Cancer in the 19th century:

The 19th century saw the birth of the scientific oncology with use of the modern microscope in studying diseased tissues. Rudolph Virchow often called the founder of cellular pathology, provided the scientific basis for modern pathologic study cancer. As Morgugni had limked autopsy findings seen with the unadded eye with clinical course of illness, so Virchow correlated microscopic pathology to illnesses.

This method not only allowed a better understanding of the damage cancer has done, but also aided the development of cancer surgery. Body tissues removed by the surgeon could now be examined and precise diagnosis could be made. The pathologist could also tell the surgeon whether the operation had completely removed.

History of cancer screening and early detection: 20th century to present.

Screening refers to tests used to find a disease, such as cancer, in people who do not have any symptoms.

First screening test to be widely used to cancer was the PAP test. The test was developed by Papanicolauu a research method in understanding menstrual cycle.

Papanicolauu soon recognised it's potential for finding cervical cancer early and presented his findings in 1923.

At first, most doctors were skeptical, and it was not untill the American Cancer society promoted the test during the early 1960s that this test became widely used. Since that time, cervical cancer incidence and mortality rates have decreased by more than 50 percent due to screening, which can detect both cervical pre-cancers and cervical cancer at an early stage.

Modern mammography methods were developed late in the 1960 s and first officially recommended by the American Cancer society in 1976. The mammogram continues to be the most reliable way to screen for breast cancer.

Future of cancer screening and early detection:

Expression profiling and proteomics. Proteomic methods are also being tested for cancer screening. For most types of cancer, measuring the amount of one protein in the blood is not very good at finding early cancers. But researchers are hopeful and that comparing the relative amounts of many proteins may be more useful, and that finding large number of certain proteins and less of others can provide accurate, useful information about the cancer treatment and its outcomes. Proteins (other types of molecules) are even found exhaled breath, which is now being tested to find out if it can show early sign of lung cancer. This is an exciting area of research and early results in lung and colorectal cancer studies have been promising.

Nanotechnology:

New technology for producing materials that form extremely tiny particles is leading to very promising imaging tests that can more accurately show the location of the tumors. It is also aiding the development of new ways to deliver drugs more specifically and effectively to cancer cells.

CHAPTER 2

INTRODUCTION OF CANCER

Cancer is a large group of diseases that can start in almost any organ or tissue of the body when abnormal cells grow uncontrollably, go beyond their usual boundaries to invade adjoining parts of the body or spread to other organs.

Cancer often has the ability to spread throughout the body. The contrast with benign tumors, which do not spread. Possible signs and symptoms include a lump, abnormal bleeding, prolonged cough, unexplained weight loss, and a change in the bowel movements. While these symptoms may indicate cancer, they can also have other cases over 100 types of cancers affect human.

Cancer is the second most common cause of death in the United States of America. But fewer people are dying of cancer now than 20 years ago. Early detection and innovative treatments are curing cancer and helping people with cancer live longer. At the same time,medical researchers are identifying independent risk factors linked to the developing cancer.

What is the difference between normal cells and cancerous cells:

Normally cells follow instructions provided by the genes.

Genes set down rules for cells to follow, such as when to start and stop growing. Cancerous cells ignore the rules that normal cell follow.

- Normal cells divide and multiply in a controlled manner. Cancerous cells multiply uncontrollably.

- Normal cells are programmed to die (apoptosis), cancerous ignore those directions.
- Normal cells for solid organs stay put. All cancerous cells are able to move around.
- Normal cells do not grow fast as cancerous cells.
- There are five broad categories indicate the tissue and blood classifications of cancer.

1 - CARCINOMA

A carcinoma is a cancer found in the body tissue known as epithelial tissue that covers or line surfaces of organs, glands, or body structures. For example, a cancer of the lining of the stomach is called a carcinoma. Many carcinomas affect organs or glands that are involved with secretion, such as breasts that produce milk.

Carcinoma accounts for 80-90 percent of all cancer cases.

- Melanoma
- Basal cell carcinoma
- Squamous cell skin cancer
- Merkel cell carcinoma.

2- SARCOMA:

Sarcoma is a malignant tumor growing from the connective tissues, such as cartilage, fat,muscle, tendons, and bones. The most common sarcoma, a Tumor on the bone, usually occurs in young adults. Examples of the sarcoma include Osteosarcoma (bone) and chondrasarcoma (cartilage).

Types of Sarcoma include:

- Soft tissue sarcoma
- Osteosarcoma
- Ewing, s sarcoma
- Chondrasarcoma.

3- LYMPHOMA

Lymphoma refers to a cancer that originates in the nodes or glands of the lymphotic system, whose job it is to produce white blood cells and clean body fluids, or in organ such as brain and breast Lymphomas are classified into two categories:

Hodgkin lymphoma and non Hodgkin lymphoma.

Types of lymphoma include:

Hodgkin,s lymphoma

Non-hodgkins lymphoma

Cutaneous lymphoma

4- LEUKEMIA

Leukemia is also known as blood cancer, is a cancer of bone marrow from producing normal red and white blood cells and platelets. White blood cells are needed to resist infection. Red blood cells are needed to prevent anemia. Platelets keep the body from easily brushing and bleeding.

Examples of leukemia include acute myelogenous leukemia, chronic myelogenous leukemia, acute lymphocytic leukemia,and chronic lymphocytic leukemia. The terms myelogenous and lymphocytic indicate the types of cells that are involved.

Types of leukemia include:

- Acute lymphocytic leukemia
- Acute myeloid leukemia
- Agnogenic myeloid leukemia
- chronic lymphocytic leukemia
- chronic myeloid leukemia
- Essential thrombocythemia (ET)
- Myelodysplastic Syndromes (MDS)

5- MYELOMA

Myeloma grows in the plasma cells of bone marrow. In some cases, the myeloma cells collect in one bone and form a single tumor, called a plasmacytoma. However, in other cases, the myeloma cells collect in many bones, forming many bone tumors. This is called multiple myeloma.

There are 18 very common cancers as given below.

Oral cancer, lung cancer, brain cancer, leukemia (blood cancer), liver cancer, pancreatic cancer, ovarian cancer, prostate cancer, stomach cancer, testicular cancer, heart cancer, breast cancer, bone cancer, colon cancer, bladder cancer, kidney cancer, skin cancer and cervical cancer.

Oral cancer:
Oral cancer is the cancer that develops in the tissues of the mouth or throat. It belongs to the large group of the cancer s called head and neck cancers. Most develop in the squamous cells found in mouth, tongue and lips.

Lung cancer:
Lung cancer is cancer that starts in the lungs and can spread to other areas of the body. The symptoms outlook, and treatment depend on the sage of the cancer and far it has spread.

Leukemia:
It refers to all cancers affecting the white blood cells. How the cancer spread can depend on the type of the leukemia and how aggressive it is.

Brain cancer:
Brain cancer is the result of cancerous cell growth. The cancer cells form tumors that can be slow growing or fast growing depending on the type of tumor.

Liver cancer: Liver cancer that occurs in the liver. Liver is the largest internal organ. It performs several critical functions to help the body eliminate waste, absorb nutrients, and heal wounds.

Pancreatic cancer:

It occurs in the tissues of pancreas, which is vital endocrine organ located behind the stomach. The pancreas plays an essential role in digestion by producing enzimes that the body needs to digest fat, carbohydrates and proteins.

Ovarian cancer:

The ovaries are small and almond shape organ located on either side the uterus. Ovarian cancer that can occur in several parts of the ovaries.

Prostate cancer:

It is most commonly diagnosed cancer in males worldwide. In the United States of America, the American Cancer society estimates that 268490 men will be newly diagnosed with this condition in 2022.

Stomach cancer:

Stomach cancer occurs when cancerous cells grow within the lining of the stomach. This type of cancer is also called gastric cancer, and it can be difficult to diagnose because most people do not show symptoms in the early stages.

Testicular cancer:

Testicular cancer is that cancer which originates in one or both testicles or testes.

Heart cancer:

Primary heart tumors are abnormal growth in the heart. They are very rare. According to the European Society of Cardiology, they are found in less than 1 out of 2000 autopsies.

Breast cancer:

Breast Cancer occurs when breast cells develop mutations and begin to divide and multiply. People may first notice a lump in the breast, discoloration, texture changes, or other symptoms.

Bone cancer:

Bone cancer occurs when a Tumor, or a typical mass of tissue forms in a bone. These are called bone sarcomas.

Colon cancer: colon cancer develops when tumorous growth form in the large intestine. It often produces no symptoms in the early stages.

Bladder cancer:

Bladder cancer is a common type of cancer that begins in the cells of the bladder. Bladder is a hollow muscular organ in the lower abdomen that stores the Urine.

Kidney cancer:

Kidney cancer is a cancer that begins in the kidneys. Kidneys are two bean shaped organs, each about size of the first.

Skin cancer:

The abnormal growth of the skin cells most often develops on the skin. But these common forms of the cancer can also occur on the areas of the skin not ordinarily exposed to the sunlight.

Cervical cancer: cervical cancer is a cancer that starts in the cells of the cervix. The cervix is the lower, narrow end of the uterus. This cervix connects uterus to the vagina (both canals). Cervical cancer usually develops slowly over the time. Before cancer appears in cervix go through the changes known se dysplasia, in which the abnormal cell begins to appear in the cervical tissue.

CHAPTER 3

ORAL CANCER

Anyone can get Oral cancer, whereas oral cancer includes the cancers of the lips or throat tissues, tongue, cheeks, floor of the mouth, hard or soft palate, sinus and throat. Let us tell you if they are not treated at the right time, they can also be fatal.

ORAL cancer is very common now, if detected early it can be easily treated. If you visit the dentist regularly, they can usually catch oral cancer in the early stages. Men have twice the risk of developing oral cancer as women. Men over the age of 50 are at greatest risk. Smoking and tobacco use is the main cause of oral cancer.

Status of mouth Cancer in India

In India, 20 people out of one lakh are suffering from oral cancer, which is 30 percent of all types of cancers. More than 5 people die every hour in India due to oral cancer.

Cancer registration is not mandatory in India, so actual figures and mortality may higher because many cases are not recorded. Most cancers in mouth are related to tobacco use, drinking alcohol, or both, and most throat cancers are caused by the Human Papilloma Virus (HPV). The incidence of HPV-Positive oral cancer has risen in the recent years.

Types of Oral cancer:

ORAL cancer can form in various parts of the mouth area. Types of oral cancer based on where they originate.

Lip cancer: As with other oral cancers, this type of typical results when the squamous cells on the surface layer of the mouth and lips begin to grow abnormally. The most new cases are diagnosed in the patients in their late 60s or early 70 s, and it often occurs on the lower lip.

Jaw cancer: Jaw cancer is a rare type of head and neck cancer. Most often, jaw cancer develops when head and neck cancer -situated in the floor of the mouth, tongue, tonsils, salivary glands or palate metastasize (spread) there.

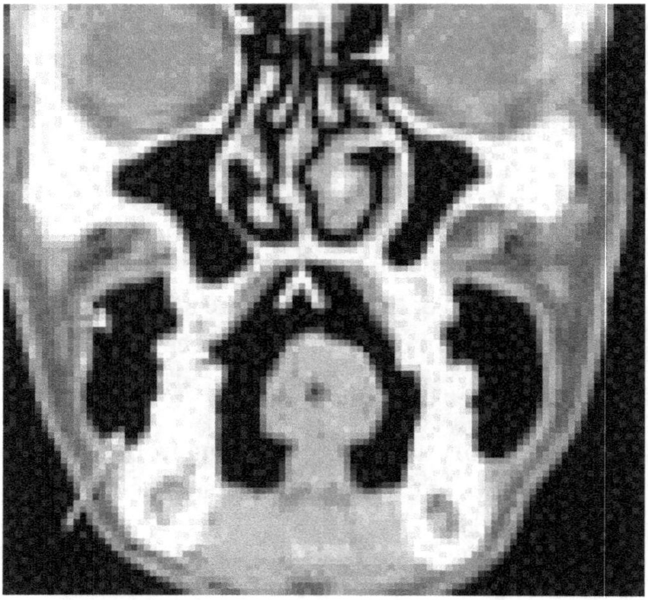

Rarely, jaw cancer may arise or its own as an Osteosarcoma, a type of cancer that forms in the bone.

Palate, cheek and other mouth Cancer: Grouped as a type of head and neck cancer, mouth Cancer (or oral cancer) may develop in the following areas.

- Gums
- Lips
- Tongue
- Inner lining of the cheek and lips (buccal mucosa)
- Floor of the mouth
- Roof of the mouth (hard palate).

Tongue cancer: It is a type of oral cancer, originates in the long flat, muscular organ known as Tongue.

Causes of oral cancer:

Tobacco and alcohol use: Tobacco of any kind, including cigarette, and electronic cigarette smoking, as well as chewing tobacco and snuff puts you at risk for the developing oral cancers. Heavy alcohol use also increases the risk.

Human Papilloma Virus (HPV): Infection with the sexually transmitted human Papilloma Virus has been linked to oral cancers.

Age: Risk increase with the age. ORAL cancers most often occur in the people over the age of 40.

Sun Exposure: Cancer of the lip can be caused by sun exposure.

Poor Nutrition: A diet low in fruits and vegetables has been linked with increased risk of oral cancer.

Genetics: people with inherited defects in certain genes have a high risk of mouth and middle throat cancer.

Symptoms of oral cancer:

Signs and symptoms of mouth Cancer may include:

- A lip or mouth sore that does not heal.
- White or redish patch on the inside of your mouth
- Loose teeth
- A growth or lump inside your mouth
- Mouth pain
- Ear pain
- Difficult or painful swallowing
- Numbness: pain or tenderness on your face and neck or in your mouth that occur without apparent cause
- Chronic bad breath

- **Oral cancer symptoms:** The following conditions all appear as patches in your mouth and throat, but they are different colors:

- **Leukemia:** These are flat white or gray patches in your mouth or throat.
- **Erythroplakia:** These are slightly raised or flat red patches might bleed when scraped
- **Erythroleukoplakia:** These patches are red and white.

Stages of Oral cancer: Oral cancers are staged using the TNM. T starts for size and location of the primary tumor, N indicates if the tumor has spread to your lymph nodes. M indicates if the tumor has metastasized, or spread to other areas of your body.

The stages for oral cavity cancer are.

- **T 1:** Tumor in your mouth measures 2 cm or less.

- T 2: The tumor is 2 cm but isn't larger than 4 cm

- T 3: The tumor is larger than 4 cm.

Treatment of oral cancer:

Most common surgeries for oral cancer:

- **Primary tumor surgery:** Healthcare providers remove tumors through your mouth or incision in your neck.
- **Glossectomy:** This is the partial or total removal of your tongue.
- **Mandibulectomy**: This the surgery for your oral cancer in your jawbone.
- **Maxillectomy:** This surgery removes part or all the bony roof of the mouth.
- **Sentinel lymph node biopsy:** This test helps healthcare providers know if cancer has spread beyond the original oral cancer
- **Neck dissection:** This surgery is done to remove lymph nodes from your neck.
- **Reconstruction:** Surgery that removes large areas of the tissue might be followed by reconstruction surgery.

Other ways to treat oral cancer:

Healthcare providers may combine surgery with other treatments, including:

- **Radiation therapy:** Radiation therapy uses strong beams of the energy to kill cancer cell or keep them from growing.
- Your healthcare provider may combine radiation therapy with other treatments.
- **Targeted therapy:** This cancer treatment uses drugs or other substances to precisely identify and attack certain type of cancer cells without hurting normal cells.
- **Monoclonal antibodies:** are immune system proteins that created in the lab and used to treat cancer.
- **Chemotherapy:** your healthcare provider may use anty - cancer drugs that kill cancer cells, including treatments that affect most parts of the body
- **Immunotherapy:** Immunotherapy is a treatment that engages your immune system to fight the disease. This treatment is sometimes called biological therapy.

Prevention of Oral cancer:

Oral cancer can be prevented and you can play an active role in preventing it.

- If your someone who smokes, chews tobacco or uses water pipe, try stopping or cutting back.

Talk to your doctor about smoking cessation programs:

- If your someone who drinks alcohol. Say to stop
- Remember your sunscreen. Use UV-AB- blocking sun screen on your face and sun block
- Get vaccinated for Human Papilloma Virus
- Eat well -balanced diet
- Have regular dental - check-ups people between 20 and 40.

Techniques of Cancer Detection or Methods for Cancer Detection:

Cancer can be detected by number of methods:

- Biopsy
- Radiography
- Blood and bone marrow tests
- ELISA (Enzyme Linked Immunoassay)
- Molecular biology techniques

Biopsy: A biopsy is a procedure to remove cells, tissue or fluid for examination by a medical pathologist, healthcare providers do biopsies when they identify areas of the concern or if you have symptoms or signs of certain conditions.

Types of biopsies

All biopsies are procedures to obtained samples of tissue and fluid, but they are done in different ways. Healthcare providers may do biopsies in medical offices or operating rooms.

Biopsy types include:

- **Bone marrow biopsy:** providers use a special biopsy needle or syringe to obtain a small sample of the bone marrow. They do bone marrow biopsies to diagnose blood cancers and other diseases.
- **Cone biopsy:** Also known as Conization or cold knife biopsy, providers do cone biopsies to remove abnormal tissue from the cervix Cone biopsy may detect cervical cancer or cervical dysplasia that could lead to cancer.
- **Excisional biopsy or incisional biopsies:** In these procedures, providers make incisions or cut in the body to remove tissue from inside body. Excisional biopsies involve removing entire lumps or suspicious areas, incisional biopsies involve taking issue samples of the lumps or suspicious areas.
- **Liquid biopsy:** This blood test detects signs of cancerous cell DNA.

- **Needle biopsy:** Providers use needle biopsies to extract cells, fluid or tissues. Your provider may order a needle biopsy if they feel unusual lump on your body or imaging tests detect potential issues.
- **Punch biopsy**: Providers use a special device to remove tissue that may be cancerous. Providers use a special device that punches a hole in your skin's surface
- **Sentinel node biopsy:** Providers do this procedure to see if cancer cells have spread from an original tumor.
- **Shave biopsy:** Providers use a razor to scrape up a small sample of skin cells to detect skin cancer.

Radiography method:

X-rays are also used in cancer diagnosis. For example, chest radiographs and mammograms are often used for early cancer detection or to see if cancer has spread to the lungs or other areas in the chest. Mammograms use X-rays to look for tumors or suspicious areas in the breasts.

- **Blood and bone marrow tests:** Bone marrow aspiration and bone marrow biopsy can show whether your bone marrow is healthy and making normal amounts of blood cells. Doctors use these procedures to diagnose and monitor blood and bone marrow diseases, including some cancers, as well as fevers of unknown origin.

Specific conditions for which the test may be performed:

- **A body-** wide fungal infection (for example disseminated coccidioidomycosis)
- A White blood cell cancer called hairy cell leukemia.
- Cancer of lymph tissue (Hodgkin or non- Hodgkin)
- Bone marrow does not make enough blood cells (aplastic anemia)

ELISA test

Stands for Enzime Linked Immunoassay. It is commonly used laboratory test to detect antibodies in the blood. An antibody is a protein produced by the body's immune system when it detects harmful substances called antigen.

Molecular biology techniques:

Molecular biology techniques include mainly: DNA cloning, DNA sequencing and synthesis, molecular hybridization, bacterial transformation and transfection, cellular screening and cellular culture, extraction of DNA, DNA polymerase, DNA dependent, reading and writing DNA etc. It is also used for infectious diseases.

CHAPTER 4
LUNG CANCER

Lung cancer is a disease caused by uncontrolled cell division in the lungs, cell divide and make more copies of themselves as a part of their normal function. But sometimes, they get changes (mutations) that cause them to keep making more of themselves when they should not. Damaged cells dividing uncontrollably create masses, or tumors, of tissue that eventually keep your organs from working properly.

Lung cancer in the name for cancers that start in your lungs- usually in the air sacs (alveoli). Cancers that start in the other places and move to your lungs are usually named for where they start. That we call it metastatic cancer.

Lung cancer, also known as Lung Carcinoma, is a malignant tumor that begins in the lungs. Lung cancer is caused by genetic damage to the DNA of cells in the airways, often caused by cigarette smoking or inhaling damaging chemicals. Damaged airways cells gain the ability to multiply unchecked causing the growth of tumor, without treatment tumors spread throughout the lung function

Early lung cancer has no symptoms and can only be detected by medical imaging. As the cancer progresses, most people experience nonspecific problems.

Types of lung cancer.

There are two main types of lung cancer, small cell lung cancer and non- small cell lung cancer. A third less common type of lung cancer is called carcinoid.

Small cell lung cancer: There are two different types of small cell lung cancer: Small cell carcinoma and mixed small cell/large cell cancer or combined small cell lung cancer.

The types of small cell lung cancer are named for kinds of cells found in the cancer and how the cells look when viewed under a microscope. Small cell lung cancer is almost always associated with cigarette smoking. Small cell lung cancer is usually treated with chemotherapy.

Small Cell Lung Cancer

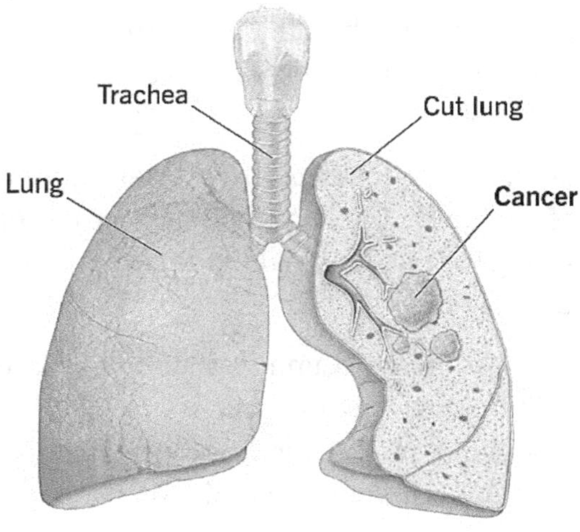

Non-small cell lung cancer:

Non-small cell is more common. It takes up 80 percent of lung cancer cases. This type of cancer usually grows and spreads to other parts of the body more slowly than small cell lung cancer does.

There three different types of non-small cell lung cancer:

1- **Adenocarcinoma:** A form of non-small cell lung cancer often found in an outer area of the lung. It develops in the cells of epithelial tissues, which line the cavities and surface of the body and form glands.

2- **Squamous cell carcinoma:** A form of non-small cell lung cancer usually found in the center of the lung next to an air tube (bronchus).

3- **Large cell carcinoma:** A form of non-small cell lung cancer that can occur in any part of the lung and tends to grow and spread faster than adenocarcinoma or squamous cell carcinoma.

Non-small cell lung cancer stages:

- **Hidden (occult):** For unknown reasons, doctors cannot identify the tumor, but cancer cells are visible in sputum or other fluid tests. Testing also suggests the cancer has not spread to nearby the lymph nodes or other places.
- **Stage 0:** The cancer is only present in the epithelial layer of cells covering the air way, with no evidence that it has gone deeper into the lung tissues, nearby lymph nodes, or any other parts of body.
- **Stage 1:** Cancer is found in lungs but has not spread to the lymph nodes or anywhere else.
- **Stage 2:** Cancer is in the lung and nearby lymph nodes.
- **Stage 3:** Cancer is in the lung and lymph nodes in the middle of the chest.

Small cell lung cancer stages:

There are two stages. In the limited stage, cancer is found in only one lung or nearby the lymph nodes on the same size of the chest.

The extensive stage means cancer has spread:

- Throughout the one lung.
- To the opposite lung
- To lymph nodes on the opposite side
- To fluid around the lung
- To bone marrow
- To distant organs.

Causes of lung cancer.

Cancers are usually caused by genetic changes (mutations) in your body's cells.

There are many factors that increase your risk of developing cancer, including the following:

- **Older age** - living longer means your body's cells may have undergone more mutations. Which may be more likely to develop cancer than younger people.
- **Smoking -** Smoking damages the cells in your lungs and increases the chance of them undergoing mutations. Smoking is a major risk factor for developing the lung cancer.
- **Family history:** Some genetic mutations that may cause cancer can be passed from parent to child.
- **Exposure of certain elements:** Significant exposure to substance such as asbestos, radon and some heavy metals may increase your risk of developing lung cancer.
- **Lung diseases:** You may have a higher chance of developing cancer if you already have lung disease such as pulmonary, fibrosis, pulmonary tuberculosis or chronic destructive pulmonary disease.

Symptoms of lung cancer:

Common symptoms of lung cancer include:

- a persistent, new cough of lung (last more than three weeks)
- a change in the cough you have had for long time.
- breathlessness
- chest or shoulder pain
- chest infection that does not go away or keeps coming back
- coughing or spitting up blood.

Other symptoms may include:

- fatigue
- unintentional weights loss
- difficulty swallowing
- hoarse voice.

Treatment of lung cancer can include:

- **Surgery, to cut out the cancer** - this includes a lobectomy where one lob of a lung is removed, a pneumonectomy, where one whole lung is removed, or a wedge resection where only part of a lung is removed.
- Radiotherapy, which damages cancer cells and stops them dividing or spreading.
- Chemotherapy, which uses strong medicine to kill the cancer cells.
- Targeted therapy, which helps your immune system see cancer cells and kill them.

Prevention of lung cancer:

You can reduce your risk of developing lung cancer by avoiding known risk factors, such as smoking and asbestos. Other risk factors, such as age and family history of lung cancer, cannot be changed.

CHAPTER 5

LEUKEMIA CANCER

Leukemia refers to all cancers affecting the white blood cells. How the cancer spreads can depend on the type of leukemia and how aggressive it is.

Leukemia starts when the DNA of single cell in your bone marrow changes (mutates) and cannot develop and function normally. Leukemia cells often behave like abnormal white blood cells. The treatment for leukemia depends on type of leukemia you have, your age and overall health, and if the leukemia has spread to other organs or tissues.

Leukemia is a cancer of blood, characterized by the rapid growth of abnormal blood cells.

The uncontrolled growth takes place in your bone marrow, where most of your body's blood is made. Leukemia cells are usually immature (still developing) white blood cells. The term leukemia comes from the Greek words for "while" (leukos) and "blood" (haima).

Unlike other cancers, leukemia doesn't generally form a mass (tumor) that shows up in imaging tests, such as X-rays or CT scans.

There are many types of leukemia. Some are more common in children, while others are more common in adults. Treatment depends on the type of leukemia and other factors.

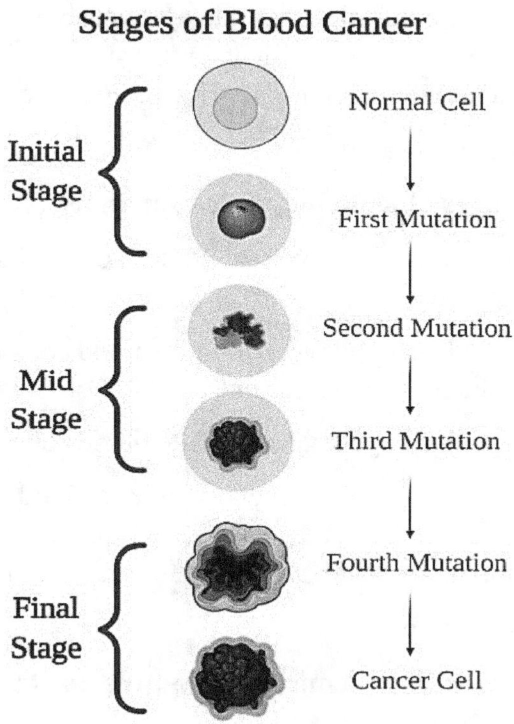

Types of leukemia:

There are 4 main types of leukemia are:

- **Acute lymphocytic leukemia:**
- This is the most common form of childhood leukemia. It can spread to your lymph nodes and Central nervous system.
- **Acute myelogenous leukemia:**
- This is the second most common form of childhood leukemia and one of the most common forms for adults.
- **Chronic lymphocytic leukemia:**
  This is the most common form of adult leukemia. Some kinds of chronic lymphocytic leukemia will be stable for years and won't need treatment. But with others, your body isn't able to create treatment.

- **Chronic myelogenous leukemia:**
  With this form, you might not have noticeable symptoms. You might not be diagnosed with it until your routine blood test. People 65 and older have higher risk of this type.

Stages of leukemia cancer:

There are 4 stages of leukemia cancer include:

Stage 1- A patient has high levels of white blood cells and enlarged lymph nodes.

Stage 2- A patient has high levels of white blood cells and is anemic. He or she may also have enlarged lymph nodes.

Stage 3- A patient has high levels of white blood cells and is anemic.

Stage 4- A patient has high levels of white blood cells and low platelets. He or she may also be anemic, have enlarged lymph nodes and have enlarged liver or spleen.

Causes of leukemia cancer:

The course of acute leukemia is unknown, but factors that put some people at higher risk are:

- exposure to intense radiation
- exposure to certain chemicals such as benzene
- viruses like the Human T- Cells leukemia virus.

Most people diagnosed with the chronic myeloid leukemia have an abnormal chromosome called Philadelphia chromosome. It has also been linked to exposure to high levels of radiation.

Symptoms of leukemia cancer:

Leukemia symptoms vary, depending on the type of leukemia. Common leukemia signs and symptoms include:

- Fever or chills
- Persistent fatigue, weakness
- Frequent or severe infections
- Losing weight without trying

- Recurrent nosebleeds
- Tiny red spots in your skin
- Excessive sweating, especially at night
- Bone pain or tenderness
- Shortness of breath
- Pale skin
- Swollen lymph nodes or stomach, an enlarged spleen or liver.
- Headache

Treatment of leukemia cancer:

Drugs (systematic therapies to treat leukemia).

Drugs that work to fight cancer in your body include:

- Chemotherapy destroys cancer cells.
- Immunotherapy helps your immune system hunt down and kill cancer.
- Targeted therapy fights cancer cells by targeting specific genetic changes in your body.

CART - T - cell therapy:

CART- T- Cell therapy, a type of immunotherapy, uses your own T-Cells to fight cancer.

Doctors may use this to treat certain types of leukemia.

Stem cell transplant to treat the leukemia.

Stem cell transplant replaces diseased cells in your body or bone marrow with healthy cells. These cells may be your own or come from the donor. Most people will first have chemo before having a stem cell transplant.

Radiation therapy

During treatment, a machine points high energy radiation beams at cancer cells to kill them or stop these from growing and spreading. Clinical trials of leukemia treatment. Talk to your cancer doctor to see if you qualify to take part in a clinical trial for new leukemia treatments Leukemia support and resources at UPMC Hillman Cancer Center.

Support services to help you your loved ones manage the physical and mental impacts of leukemia include:

- Counseling
- Leukemia support groups.
- Access to resources near you.

Cancer cares close to home.

UPMC Hillman Cancer Center has more than 2000 cancer experts and 70 locations in Pennsylvania, Ohio, Maryland and Western New York. And as one of the largest community cancer networks in the U.S.

Prevention of leukemia cancer.

There is no confirm way to prevent the leukemia. Still, it may be possible to help reduce the risk for this type of cancer by making life certain life style changes and following healthy habits, including:

- **Don't smoke:** current smokers should seek help to quit. There are lots of free cessation programs available online or in the local community. Keep trying and find what works.
- Keep a healthy weight

Lose weight if needed

- Avoid or lower exposure to chemicals that they may raise the risk for leukemia, such as benzene and formaldehyde
- Lower exposure to the pesticides
- Stay physically active and follow a healthy diet. Both these lifestyle elements have been proven to reduce the cancer risk in general.

CHAPTER 6

BRAIN CANCER

Brain cancer can be malignant (cancerous) or benign (noncancerous) and can affect children and adults. But whether they are cancerous or not, brain tumor can impact your function if they grow large enough to press on surrounding tissues. There are several treatment options for brain tumors.

Brain cancers include Primary brain tumors, which start in the brain and almost nerve spread to other parts of the body, and secondary tumors (metastases), which are caused by cancers that began in another part of the body.

Cancerous brain tumors cause symptoms that get worse quickly. Cancerous brain tumors also are called brain cancers or malignant brain tumors.

They cause symptoms that come on suddenly. They get worse in a matter of days.

These are more than 40 major types of brain tumors, which are grouped into two main types:

- benign-slow-growing and unlikely to spread. Common types are meningiomas, neuromas, pituitary tumors and carciniopharyngiomas.
- malignant - cancerous and able to spread other parts of the brain or spinal cord. Common types include astrocytomas, oligodendrogliomas and mixed gliomas.

It is estimated that more than 1900 people were diagnosed with brain cancer in 2023. The average age at diagnosis is 59 years old.

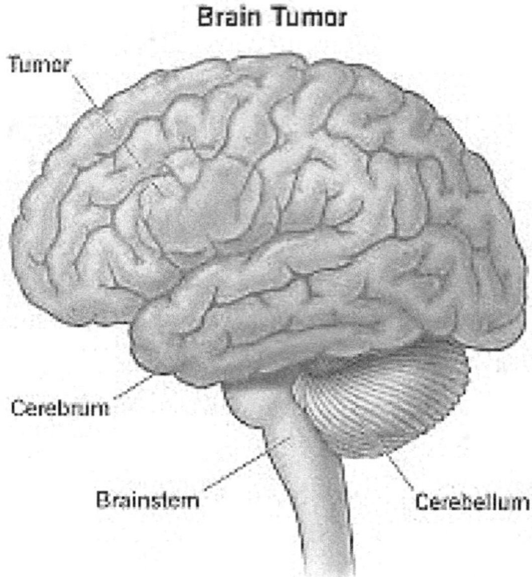

Causes of brain cancer

Generally speaking, brain tumors are a result of genetic mutations in healthy cells. These genetic mutations cause healthy brain cells to grow and divide much faster than normal, while also preventing them from the dying off when natural life cycle complete.

This rapid buildup of Cells in what form a tumor.

Although the exact causes of primary brain cancer are not fully understood, there are several factors that have been attributed to an increased risk for developing it.

Brain cancer risk factors:

Researchers have discovered several brain cancer risk factors, which are traits can make a person more susceptible to tumors of brain and spinal cord. That's not to say that the people who have one (or more) of these traits will develop cancer. Many people have several of these characteristics and live perfectly healthy lives.

Additionally, brain tumors can develop in people who have no known risk factors at all. For the most part, the risk factors are used to identify individuals who should closely monitor their health and report any potential brain cancer symptoms to a physician.

Brain cancer risk factors you can change:

Research suggests the following controllable factors may influence brain cancer risk.

- **Radiation therapy:** exposure to ionizing radiation- specifically when it is delivered to the head or neck may increase the likelihood of developing brain cancer.
- **Environmental exposure:** There may be a link between brain cancer and frequent exposure to certain chemicals found in the

pesticides, fertilizer, solvents, vinyl chloride and oil products although more research on this subject is needed.

Brain cancer risk factors you can't change:

Most risk factors for brain cancer can't control. These include:

- **Age-** brain cancer occur at any age but it is most common in children and older adults.
- **Biological sex-** Generally speaking, men are more likely to develop brain cancer than women.
- Family Medical history Around 5 percent of brain tumors can be linked to the familial syndrome like neurofibromatosis, Li-Fraumeni syndrome, tuberculosis sclerosis and Vin Hippel-lindau disease.
- **Weakened immune system -** Having a compromised immune system from congenital or acquired factors (such as HIV or AIDS) can leave a person more susceptible to certain types of brain cancer.

Brain cancer grades:

Brain cancer is usually graded rather than staged. The brain tumor grading system features four distinct grades and provides your care team with an understanding of how the tumor grows. This process helps doctors match brain cancer treatments to individual needs.

Brain cancer is categorized into 4 grades. They are:

Grade 1 Brain cancer: The tumor grows slowly and rarely spreads into nearby tissue. It may be possible to completely remove the tumor with Surgery.

Grade 2 brain cancer: The tumor grows slowly but may spread into nearby tissues or reoccur.

Grade 3 Brain cancer: The tumor grows quickly, is likely to spread into nearby tissues, and tumor cells look very different from normal cells.

Grade 4 Brain Cancer: The tumor grows and spread very quickly, and tumor cells do not look like normal Cells.

Brain metastasis: secondary brain tumors, which have spread to the brain from another location in the body, are much more common that primary brain tumors. These tumors also becoming increasingly more common as individuals do better with cancer treatment and live longer, giving the original cancer the opportunity to spread the brain Some cancers that commonly spread to the brain are lung, breast, colon, kidney, Melanoma, thyroid and uterine.

Lung cancer is the most common form of brain metastasis. In fact, lung cancer staging often involves a brain scan.

Symptoms of brain cancer: Early signs of brain cancer may include:

A headach that changes depending on the time of day and position of the head and gets worse overtime.

Common symptoms of brain cancer may also include:

- Nausea or vomiting
- Memory loss
- Muscles weakness
- speech difficulty
- Mood or personality changes
- Unexplained tiredness

- Changes in the Menstrual cycle
- Impotence or infertility
- Overproduction or unproduction of breast milk
- Cushing's syndrome (a condition marked by weight gain)
- High blood pressure
- Diabetes
- Brushing

Some patients may not feel right cognitively, or have visual, speech or coordination problems. The symptoms may be subtle or develop gradually.

Brain cancer treatment:

Treatment of brain cancer is usually complex. Most treatment plans involve several doctors.

- Neurosurgeons
- Oncologists
- Radiation Oncologists
- Your primary data: Team may also include a dietician, a social worker, a physical therapist, and other therapists.

The most widely treatments are surgery, radiation therapy, and chemotherapy. In most cases more than one of these used on:

- Types of tumor
- Size and location of the tumor
- Your Age and overall health
- The risk of particular treatment
- Other medical problems you have
- The treatment you most prefer

Brain cancer surgery: Common types of surgery include:

- Craniotomy This is the surgery most often used to remove a brain tumor.
- Neuroendoscopy. The surgeon makes a small whole in the skull or goes through the nose or mouth, depending on the location of the tumor.

- Radiation therapy for brain cancer. Radiation therapy uses high energy rays to kill the tumor cells, stopping them from growing spreading.

Radiation can be given in the following ways:

- **External radiation.**
  The treatments are usually given 5 days. Each treatment takes only few minutes.
- **Internal or implant radiation.**
  Uses a tiny radioactive capsule that is placed inside the tumor. Radiation from the capsule destroys the tumor.
- **Stereotactic radiosurgery.**
  Destroys the brain tumor without opening the skull.

Chemotherapy for brain cancer:

Chemotherapy is the use of powerful medicines to kill the tumor cells.

- You may get single medicine or a combination of them.
- Chemotherapy is given by mouth or IV. Some medications are through the shunt put in place to drain excess fluid from the brain.

Prevention of brain cancer:

You can reduce your risk of developing a brain tumor by avoiding environmental hazards, such as smoking, an excessive exposure of the radiation.

It's important to understand your risk factors to maintain good health.

CHAPTER 7

LIVER CANCER

Primary cancer is a disease in which malignant (cancer) cells form in the tissues of the liver. Cancer that forms in other parts of the body and spreads to the liver is not primary liver cancer. The liver is one of the largest organs in the body. It has two lobes and fills the upper right side of the abdomen inside the rib cage.

When cancer starts in the liver, it is called liver cancer. Liver cancer is a cancer that's found anywhere in the liver.

Primary liver cancer is an uncommon but serious type of cancer that begins in the liver.

This is a separate condition from secondary cancer, which occurs when cancer that first develops in another part of the body spreads to the liver.

Unlike other cells in your body, cancer cells can break away from the primary site, or where the cancer began.

The cells can travel to other areas of your body through the blood streams or lymphotic system. When they reach other organs or tissues, they can begin to grow there.

Causes of liver cancer:

Risk factors for liver cancer development include:

Type 2 diabetes: People with diabetes especially if they also have hepatitis or regularly consume a lot of alcohol, are more likely to develop liver cancer.

Liver Cancer Development

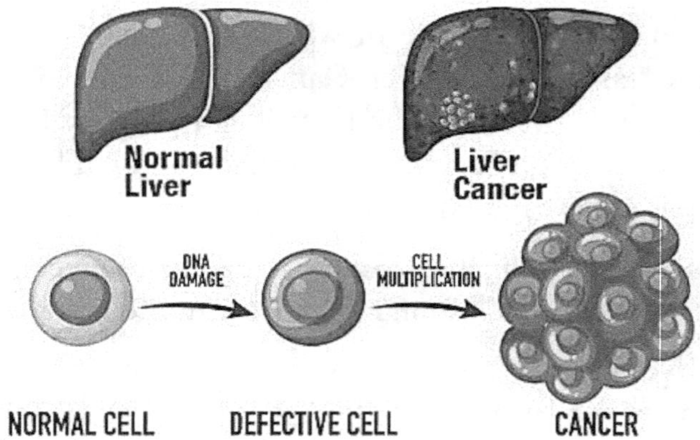

Family history: If someone's mother, father, brother, or sister has had liver cancer, they have higher risk of developing the disease themselves.

Heavy alcohol use:

Consuming more than six alcoholic drinks every day for an extended period can lead to cirrhosis. This, in turn, increases the risk of liver cancer.

Long term exposure to aflatoxins: A particular fungus creates a substance called aflatoxin. When mold grows on the following crops, it can lead to the presence of aflatoxins:

- Wheat
- Corn
- Nuts
- Soybeans
- Peanuts

The risk of liver cancer only increases following long-term exposure to aflatoxins. These substances are less of a worry in industrialized nations where manufacturers regularly test for aflatoxins.

Low immunity: People with weakened immune systems, such as HIV, or AIDS have a risk of liver cancer. That is five times greater than other healthy quality individuals.

Obesity: Being obese raises the risk of developing many cancers. In people who go on to develop liver cancer, obesity can contribute to cirrhosis and fatty liver disease.

Smoking: Both former and current smokers have a higher risk of liver cancer than people who have never smoked.

Individuals who have a high risk for liver cancer should have regular screening for liver cancer. They include those with:

- hepatitis B or C alcohol related cirrhosis
- cirrhosis due to hemochromatosis, a disorder that involves deposits of iron salts in the body tissue.

Liver cancer becomes very difficult to cure if a doctor diagnoses it at a later stage.

Screening is the only effective way of catching liver cancer early because symptoms of the early-stage liver cancer are either subtle or nonexistent.

Stages of liver cancer:

Stages of liver cancer based on 3 factors.

- **Tumor (T):** This is an assessment of how large the cancer is and if there are multiple tumors
- **Lymph nodes (N):** This notes whether or not the cancer has spread into your nearby lymph nodes or organs.

Stage 4 A: Liver cancer consists of:

- a single tumor or multiple tumors of any size (any T)
- cancer that has spread to your nearby lymph nodes (N)
- cancer that has not spread to your distant organs and tissues (M1)

When it has metastasized, liver cancer is more likely to spread to certain areas. These include your:

- lungs
- bones
- brain
- abdominal glands

Symptoms of liver cancer.

Most people do not have signs and symptoms in the early stages of the primary liver cancer. When signs and symptoms do appear, they may include:

- losing weight without trying
- loss of appetite
- upper abdominal pain
- nausea and vomiting
- General weakness.
- abdominal swelling
- yellow discoloration of your skin and the whites of your eyes (jaundice)
- white chalky stools
- fatigue

Dark color urine does not make it bold.

Treatment of liver cancer make it bold.

Surgery: Operations used to treat liver cancer include:

Surgery to remove tumor: In certain conditions doctor recommends an operation to remove liver cancer a small portion of healthy liver tissue that it surrounds it if tumor is small and liver function is good

Liver transplant surgery: During liver transplant surgery, your diseased liver is removed and replaced with the healthy liver from a donor. Liver transplant surgery is only option for a small percentage of people with early-stage liver cancer

Radiation therapy: Radiation therapy might be an option if other treatments are not possible or if they have not help. For advanced liver cancer radiation therapy might have control symptoms.

Targeted therapy: Many targeted drugs are available for treating advanced liver cancer. Some targeted therapies only work in people whose cancer cells have certain genetic mutations.

Immunotherapy: Immunotherapy uses your immune system to fight cancer.

Immunotherapy treatments are reserved for people with advanced liver cancer.

Chemotherapy:

The chemotherapy uses drugs to kill the rapidly growing cells, including cancer cells. Chemotherapy can be administered through a vein in your arm, in pills form or both.

Chemotherapy is sometimes used to treat advanced liver cancer.

Prevention of liver cancer: The following are protective factors for liver cancer:

- Getting the hepetitis B Vaccine
- Getting treatment for chronic hepetitis B infection
- Reducing exposure to aflatoxin B1.

CHAPTER 8

PANCREATIC CANCER

Pancreatic occurs when maglinant cells develop in the part of the pancreas. This may affect how the pancreas works, including the functioning of the exocrine or endocrine glands. Pancreatic cancer can occur any part of the pancreas, about 70 percent of pancreatic cancers are located in the head of the pancreas.

Pancreatic is caused by changes in the DNA of the pancreatic organ. The mutations in pancreatic cells leads to uncontrolled growth and reproduction of pancreatic cells and formation of masses, or it can cause normal cells to die and fail to function. If left untreated, it can spread to other organs. The pancreatic cancer most often arises from cells in the duct that secretes enzymes into the digestive tract. Sometimes tumors arising from the hormone - producing cells of the pancreas can also be seen.

Although the causes of pancreatic cancer are not clearly known, there are some risk factors for pancreatic cancer, just like any other disease.

Catching pancreatic cancer early is challenging because patients rarely experience the signs of pancreatic cancer until the disease has progressed or spread

Types of pancreatic cancer:

Pancreatic cancer types can be divided into two larger categories.

1. Exocrine pancreatic cancer.
2. Neuroendocrine pancreatic cancer.

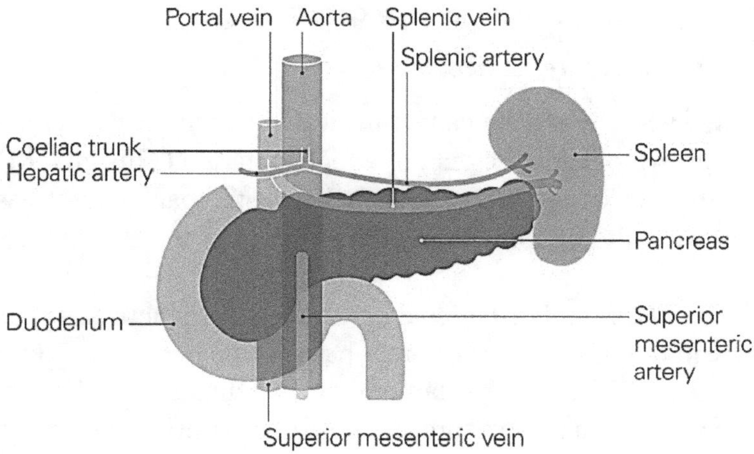

1. **Exocrine pancreatic cancer:** various types of exocrine pancreatic cancers make up more than 95 percent of all the cancers of the pancreas. They include:

- **Adenocarcinoma:** This cancer occurs in the lining of the duct in the pancreas.
- **Squamous cell carcinoma:** Studies have reported that it has a very bad prognosis due to most cases being discovered after metastasis.

Adenosquamous carcinoma: These tumors show characteristics of both ductal adenocarcinoma and squamous cell carcinoma.

Colloid carcinoma: Pancreatic colloid tumor consists of malignant cell that float in a gelatinous substance called mucin, it is not likely to spread and easier to treat than other pancreatic cancers. It also has much better prognosis.

2. **Neuroendocrine pancreatic cancer:** Pancreatic neuroendocrine tumors devlop from cells in the endocrine glands of the pancreas, which secretes the homones insulin and glucagon into the bloodstream to regulate blood sugar. Also known as endocrine or

islet cell tumors, neuroendocrine cancers are rare, making up less than 5 percent of all pancreatic cancer cases.

Stages of pancreatic cancer.

- **Stage 0:** Refers to the cancer in situ, in which the cancer has not yet grown outside the duct in which it started (This NO. MO)
- **Stage 1A:** Tumor is 2cm or smaller in the pancreas. It has not spread to the lymph nodes or other parts of the body (T 1, NO, MO)
- **Stage 1B:** A tumor larger than 2cm in the pancreas. It has not spread to lymph nodes or other parts of the body (T2, NO, MO)
- **Stage 2 A:** The tumor is larger than 4cm and extends beyond the pancreas. It has not spread to nearby arteries, veins, lymph nodes, or other parts of the body (T3, NO, MO)
- **Stage 2B:** A tumor of any single size has not spread to nearby arteries or veins. It has spread to 1to3 regional lymph nodes but no to other parts of the body (T1, T2 or T3: N1; MO)

Stage 3. Either of these conditions:

- A number of any size that has spread to 4 or more regional lymph nodes but not to nearby arteries veins or other parts of the body (T1, T2 or T3, N2, MO)
- A tumor that has spread to nearby arteries and veins and may have spread to regional lymph nodes. It has not spread other parts of the body (T4, any N, MO)

Stage 4 Any tumor has spread to other parts of the body (any T, any N, M1)

Symptoms of pancreatic cancer.

Pancreatic cancer symptoms may include

- Jaundice (Yellowing of your skin)
- Dark urine
- light colour stool
- Upper abdominal pain
- Itchy skin

- Nausea and vomiting
- Gas or bloating
- lack of appetite
- Blood cots
- Weight loss
- Diabetes.

Causes of pancreatic cancer:

Who is likely to get pancreatic cancer. Anyone can get pancreatic cancer. It is not very clear what causes it. You might be more likely to get if you:

- Over the age of 65. It is not very common in people under 40
- Have certain medical conditions, such as chronic pancreatitis
- There is history of pancreatic cancer in your family

Many pancreatic cancers are also linked to your lifestyles.

Treatment of pancreatic cancer:

Surgery: If the cancer is localized at the time of diagnosis, it may be possible to iliminate the cancer by removing all or parts of the pancreas are.

- **Whipple procedure:** A surgeon removed the pancreas head and sometimes the whole pancreas, along with a portion of the stomach, duodenum, lymph nodes, and other tissues.

- Complications include leaking, infections, bleeding, and stomach problems.

- **Distal pancreatectomy:** The surgeon removed part of the pancreas usually the spleen as well.

- **Total pancreatectomy:** In total pancreatectomy, the surgeon removed the entire pancreas and spleen.

- **Palliative surgery:** A surgion can create a bypass, so that bile can continue to flow from the liver. This can minimize pain and digestive systems.

- **Embolization:** In embolization, a healthcare professional will inject into an artery a substance that stops blood from reaching the cancer cells without the blood supply, these cells will die.

Chemotherapy: Chemotherapy is often used after surgery to kill many cancer cells that might remain.

When the cancer is advanced and spread to other parts of the body, chemotherapy can help control it Chemotherapy might help relieve symptoms, such as pain

When cancer is treated with high power medicine that we call it chemotherapy.

Radiotherapy: When surgery isn't an option, the radiation therapy might be the first treatment.

Immunotherapy: Immunotherapy might be option if your pancreatic cancer has specific DNA changes that would make it cancer likely to these treatments.

Prevention of pancreatic cancer.

- A typical American diet, high in fat and smoked other processed. meats, has been associated with pancreatic cancer in some but not at all studies.
- Health diet rich in the fresh fruits and vegetables to be used
- Protein, high fat diet were consistently found to develop pancreatic cancer, however, laboratory data doesn't necessarily apply to the people.
- Do not smoke
- Do exercise.

CHAPTER 9

OVARIAN CANCER

The ovaries are small, almond shaped organs located on either side of the uterus. Eggs are produced in the ovaries. Ovarian Cancer can occur in several different parts of the ovary.

Ovarian cancer is the growth of cells that forms in the ovaries. The cells multiply quickly and can invade and destroy healthy body tissue.

The female reproductive system contains two ovaries, one on each side of the uterus. The ovaries - each about size of an almond - produce eggs (ova) as well as the hormones estrogen and progesterone.

Ovarian cancer is sometimes difficult to detect because symptoms often do not develop until later stages. Healthcare providers treat ovarian cancer with surgery, chemotherapy and cancer treatments

Ovarian cancers come in a variety of different tumor types and subtypes. The most common tumor type is serious adenocarcinoma, and the common subtype is serious adenocarcinomas are high grade tumors.

Types of ovarian Cancer.

There are three types of ovarian Cancer:

- **Epithelial ovarian cancer:** These are the most common types of ovarian cancer. About 85 to 90 percent of these cancers involve the cells that over the outer surface of the ovary. They commonly spread first to the lining and organs of the pelvis and abdomen and then to other parts of the body. Nearly 70 percent of women with this type of ovarian cancer are diagnosed in the advanced stages.

- 2 - **Germ cell tumors:** These make up less than 2 percent of all ovaries cancers.

They begin in the reproductive cells that are a woman's "egg".

90 percent of patients with Germ cell tumors survive 5 years after diagnosis. Teenagers and women in their 20s are more likely to develop this type of ovarian cancer.

3 - **Stromal cell tumors:** These represent about 1 percent of all the ovarian cancers. They form in the tissues that support the ovaries. This type of cancer is often found in the early stages. Vaginal bleeding is one the most common.

Stages of ovarian cancer:

Stage 1 ovarian cancer: Stage one cancer means the cancer is only in the ovaries. Surgery is the main treatment. Some women need chemotherapy.

Stage II Endometrial Cancer

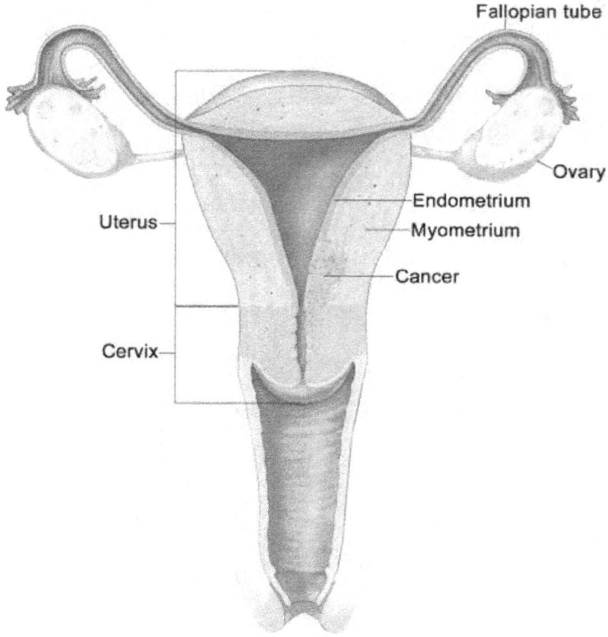

Stage 2 ovarian cancer: Stage 2 ovarian cancer means the cancer has grown outside the ovaries and growing within the pelvis. The treatment is surgery and chemotherapy.

Stage 3 ovarian cancer: Stage 3 ovarian cancer has spread outside the pelvis into the abdominal cavity or to lymph nodes. Treatment is surgery and chemotherapy.

Stage 4 ovarian cancer: Stage 4 ovarian cancer has spread to other body organs some distance away from the ovaries, such as the liver or lungs. The main treatment surgery and chemotherapy.

Causes of ovarian cancer: Some factors that can increase your risk of ovarian cancer include:

- Age (risk increases for women over 50).
- Family history of ovarian cancer, breast or bowel cancer.
- Changes in the genes BRCA 1 or BRCA 2.
- Being of Ashkenazi Jewish descent.
- Early onset of periods (before 12 years) and late menopause Women who have not had children or had their first child of 35.
- Using oestrogen only hormone replacement therapy or fertility treatment.

Symptoms of ovarian cancer: There are often no signs of ovarian cancer, however you may have one or more of the following symptoms:

- Abdominal bloating
- Difficulty eating or feeling full quickly
- Frequent or urgent urination
- Back, abdominal or pelvic pain
- Constipation or diarrhea
- Menstrual irregularities
- Tiredness
- Indigestion
- pain during intercourse
- Unexplained weight gain or weight loss.

Treatment of ovarian cancer:

Types of treatment:

Chemotherapy: Chemotherapy uses anti - cancer drugs to destroy the cancer cells. Most women will have chemotherapy after surgery to destroy any remaining cancer cells.

Some women will have chemotherapy before surgery with the aim to shrink tumors and make them easier to remove.

Chemotherapy is usually given as combination of two drugs or sometimes as a single drug, delivered as liquid into vein.

Radiation therapy: Radiation therapy can used to treat the pelvis or other sites of cancer that have spread. It may be used on its own or after chemotherapy.

Prevention of ovarian cancer:

Sometimes a woman may want to consider having both ovaries and fallopian tubes removed (called a bilateral salpingo - oophorectomy) to reduce the risk of ovarian cancer before cancer is even suspected. If the ovary is removed to prevent ovarian cancer, the surgery is called risk - reducing or prophylactic.

CHAPTER 10

PROSTATE CANCER

Prostate cancer is the most commonly diagnosed cancer in the males worldwide. In the United States, the American Cancer society estimates that 268490 men will be newly diagnosed within this condition in 2022.

Prostate cancer is a cancer that occurs in the prostate. The prostate is a small walnut- shaped galand in males that produces the seminal fluid that naurishes and transport sperm

Prostate cancer is one of the most common types of cancer. Many prostate cancers grow slowly and are confined to the prostate gland, where they may not cause serious harm. However, while some types of prostate cancer

grow slowly and may need minimal or even no treatment, other

Types are aggressive and spread quickly.

Types of prostate cancer: Main types of the prostate cancer are as given below:

Adenocarcinoma: Adenocarcinoma may occur almost anywhere in the body. They form in the glandular epithelial cells that line the insides of the organs and secrete mucus, digestive juices or other fluids. In the prostate, adenocarcinoma is called glandular prostate cancer.

Main subtypes of adenocarcinoma of prostate (conventional adenocarcinoma): This cancer accounts for vertually all prostatic adenocarcinomas. Acini cells line the prostate's fluid - screening in the back (periphery) of the prostate near rectum and may be felt during a doctor's digital rectal exam. The disease increases PSA levels.

Prostatic ductal adenocarcinoma (PDA): This cancer is rare but more aggressive form of adenocarcinoma. It develops in the cells lining the tubes ducts of the prostate galand. When it occurs, it frequently deveps along with acinar adenocarcinoma. This cancer type doesn't necessarily increase PSA levels, making it harder to detect.

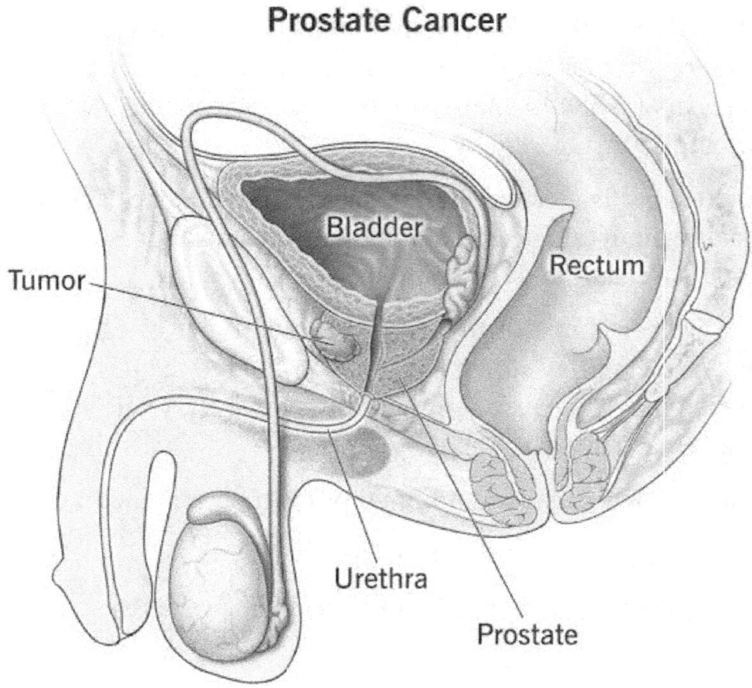

Stages of prostate cancer.

TNM stages staging system: Doctors use the results from diagnostic tests and scans to answer these questions.

- **Tumor (T):** How large is the primary tumor? Where it is located?
- **Node (N):** Has the tumor spread to the lymph nodes? If so, where and how many? Lymph nodes are small, bean shaped organs that help fight infection.

- **Metastasis (M):** Has the cancer spread to other parts of the body? If so, where and how much?

The results are combined to determine the stage of the cancer for each person.

There are 5 stages: stage 0 (zero) and stage 1 through 4. The stage provides a common way of describing the cancer, so the doctors can work together to plan the best treatment.

Causes of prostate cancer: The most common risk factors include:

- **Age:** Risk increase as you get older. You are more likely to get diagnosed if you are over 50. About 60 percentage of prostate cancers occur in people older than 65.
- **Face and ethnicity:** You are at greater risk if you are black or of African ancestry. You are more likely to develop prostate cancers that are more likely to spread. You are also at greater risk of prostate cancer forming before age 50.
- **Family history of prostate cancer:** You are 2 to 3 times more likely to get prostate cancer if a close family member has it.
- **Genetics:** You are at greater risk if you have Lynch syndrome or if you inherited muted (changed) genes associated with increased breast cancer risk.

Some studies have identified other prostate cancer risk factors, but the evidence is mixed. Other potential risk factors include:

- Smoking
- Prostatitis
- Having BMI (Body Mass Index) greater than 30 (having obesity)
- Sexually transmitted Infection (STI)
- Exposure to agent Orange (a chemical used during the Vietnam war)

Symptoms for prostate cancer: prostate cancer may cause no signs or symptoms in its early stage.

Prostate cancer that's more advanced may cause signs and symptoms such as:

- Trouble urinating
- Decreased force in the stream of urine
- Blood in the Urine
- Blood in semen
- Bone pain
- losing weight without trying
- Erectile dysfunction.

Treatment of prostate cancer: prostate Cancer is the most common cancer in men. If diagnosed it in early stage it is completely cureable.

In the early stages, there are no symptoms of prostate cancer, and is only the test to diagnose prostate cancer is a simple blood test called PSA. Any PSA value above 4 ng/ml to rule out prostate cancer.

Robotic Radical Prostatectomy: Robotic surgery is the most advanced treatment of prostate cancer. In this technology, by the use of robotic Arms, we take out the whole prostate through small holes in the body. In the robotic surgery by Dr Ashish Sabharwal. There is minimal pain, minimal blood loss, and no need for blood transfusion or ICU stay, early return to normal activity. We do nerve sparing Robotic radical Prostatectomy. So there is early return of urinary control and preservation of erections.

Prevention of Prostate cancer:

Add citrus to your diet: Eating fresh fruits in an important part of balanced diet. It's also possible that it may lower your risk of prostate cancer.

A 2017 study found that people who consumed the highest amount of fruit, especially citrus, had a small reduction in their risk of prostate cancer.

Some examples of citrus fruits to consider trying out are:

- Oranges
- Grapefruit
- Lemons
- Limes
- Tangerines
- Mandarin oranges
- Kumquats
- Yuzu

It is important note that grapefruit can interact with some type of medication. If take prescription medications are unsure whether you can have grapefruits, be sure to talk with your doctor first.

Limit saturated fat:

A 2014 review of research may be linked between saturated fats and animal fats and an increase prostate cancer risk.

Whenever possible, replace saturated and animal fats with plant-based fats Olive oil instead of butter.

Fruits instead of candy.

Fresh vegetables instead of prepacked foods.

Nuts or seeds instead of cheese.

Make time for exercise.

CHAPTER 11

STOMACH CANCER

Stomach cancer occurs when cancerous cells grow within the lining of the stomach. This type of cancer is also called gastric cancer, and can be difficult to diagnose because most people typically do not show symptoms in the earliest stages. It is common worldwide but rare in the U.S. Common stomach symptoms like unexplained weight loss and stomach pain often do not appear in the early stages.

Cancer cells grow out of control in your stomach. Cancer can form anywhere in your stomach. In the U.S. most cases of stomach cancer involve abnormal cell growth in place of where your stomach meets your esophagus (gastroesophageal junction). In other countries, where gastric cancer is more common, cancer usually forms in the main part of the stomach.

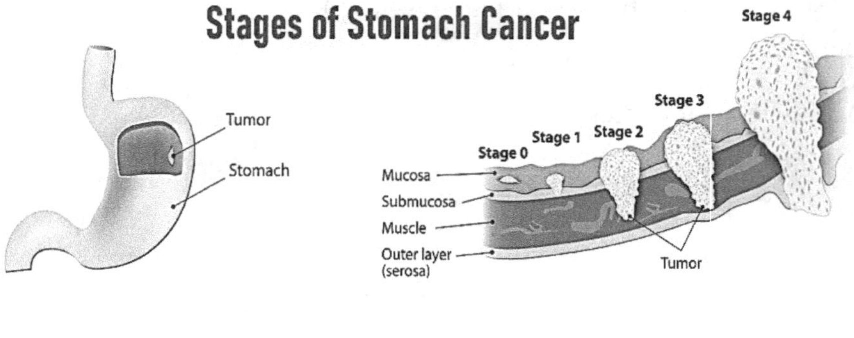

About 95 percent of the time, stomach cancer starts in the stomach lining and progresses slowly. Untreated, it can form a mass (tumor) and grow deeper into your stomach walls. The tumor may spread to nearby organs like your liver and pancreas

Stages of stomach cancer:

Stage 0: Stage 0 Refers to carcinoma in situ. This means that abnormal cells are found in the mucosa. These abnormal cells may become cancer and spread into nearby normal tissue.

Stage 1 is divided into stages 1 A and 1B.

- In stage 1A
- Cancer has formed in the mucosa and may have spread to the submucosa.
- In stage 1B
- Cancer has formed in the mucosa and may have spread to the submucosa and has spread to 2 or 2 nearby lymph nodes, or - Cancer has formed in the mucosa and has spread to the muscle layer.

Stage 2: stage 2 is divided into 2 A and 2B

- **Stage 2 A:** Cancer may have spread to the submucosa and has spread to 3 to 6 nearby lymph nodes; or Cancer has spread to the muscles layer and to 1 or 2 nearby lymph nodes; or Cancer has spread to submucosa.

In stage 2B:

- Cancer may have spread to the submucosa and has spread to 7 to 15 nearby lymph nodes; or

- Cancer has spread to the muscle layer and to 3 to 6 lymph nodes; or

- Cancer to the submucosa and to 1 or 2 nearby lymph nodes; or

- Cancer has to the serosa

Stage3: Stomach cancer tag 3 is divided into stages 3 A, 3B,3C.

Stage 4: In stage 4 cancer has spread to other parts of the body, such as lungs, liver, distant lymph nodes, and tissues that lines the abdomen walls.

The metastatic tumor is the same type of cancer as the primary tumor. **For example,** if the stomach cancer spread to the lung, the cancer cells in the lung are actually stomach cancer cells. The disease is called metastatic stomach cancer, not lung cancer.

Types of stomach cancer:

- Adenocarcinoma. Adenocarcinoma stomach cancer starts in cells that produce mucus.
- Gastrointestinal stromal tumors (GIST). GIST starts in the special nerve cells that found in the wall of the stomach and other digestive organs.
- Carcinoid tumors.
- Lymphoma.

Causes of stomach cancer.

- Smoking
- Being overweight or obese
- A diet high in smoked, pickled or salty foods
- Drinking of alcohol regularly
- Stomach surgery for an ulcer
- Type A blood.
- Certain genes
- H. Pylori bacteria (infection)

Symptoms of stomach cancer: As stomach tumors grow, you may have more serious symptoms, such as:

- Stomach pain
- Blood in your stool
- Vomiting
- Weight loss for no reason
- Trouble swallowing
- Yellow eyes or skin
- Swelling in your stomach
- Constipation or diarrhea
- Weakness or feeling tired
- Heartburn.

Treatment of stomach cancer:

1. **Endoscopic mucosal resection:** This is a procedure that uses an endoscope to remove carcinoma in situ and earlystage cancer from the lining of the digestive tract. An endocsope is a thin and a lens and tools to remove the tissue

- **Surgery:** goal of surgery for stomach cancer which is called gastric cancer, is to remove all of the cancers. For small stomach cancer, surgery might be first treatment. Other treatments might be used first if stomach cancer grows deeper into stomach walls or spread to the lymph nodes.

Operations used to treat stomach cancer include:

- **Removing small cancer from the stomach lining:** This procedure is called an endoscopic mucosal resection. It might be an option for treating stage 1 cancer that is growing on the inner lining of the stomach cancer
- **Removing part of the stomach:** It might be an option if your stomach cancer is located in the parts of the stomach nearest to the small intestine.
- **Removing the entire stomach**: Total gastrectomy is a treatment for cancer in the part of the stomach that closest to the esophagus
- **Removing lymph nodes to look for cancer:** Surgeon may remove lymph nodes in your belly to test them for cancer.
- **Surgery to relieve symptoms**: This might be an option if the cancer is advanced and other treatments have not helped

2- **Chemotherapy:** This is a drug treatment that uses chemicals to kill cancer cells. Types of chemotherapy include:

- **Chemotherapy that travels through your whole body:** This is called systematic chemotherapy. Medicine can be given through vein or taken pills form
- **Chemotherapy that only goes in the belly:** After the surgeon removed the stomach cancer, the chemotherapy medicines are put directly into the belly.

Radiation therapy: Radiation therapy might be used after surgery if they can't be removed completely. Giving radiation after surgery is called adjuvant radiation.

Radiation can help relieve stomach cancer symptoms if the cancer is advanced.

3- Immunotherapy:

Immunotherapy is sometimes used to treat advanced cancer. This might include stage 4 Stomach cancer or cancer comes back after treatment.

Palliative care: When palliative care is used along with all the other appropriate treatments, people with cancer may feel better and live longer.

Prevention of stomach cancer: Diet, nutrition, body weight, physical activity, and alcohol use. Being over Weight or obese increases the risk of some types of stomach cancer. So getting to and staying at healthy weight might lower your risk. Getting regular physical activity might also help lower your risk of stomach cancer.

CHAPTER 12

TESTICULAR CANCER

Testicular cancer which is the cancer that originates in one or both testicles or testes.

Testicular cancer happens when cells in the testicles grow to form tumor. This is rare, more than 90 percent of testicular cancers begin in the germ cells, which produce sperm. These two types of germ cell cancers.

Seminoma can grow slowly and respond very well to radiation and chemotherapy.

Non - seminal can grow more quickly and can be less responsive to those of treatments.

Testicular cancer

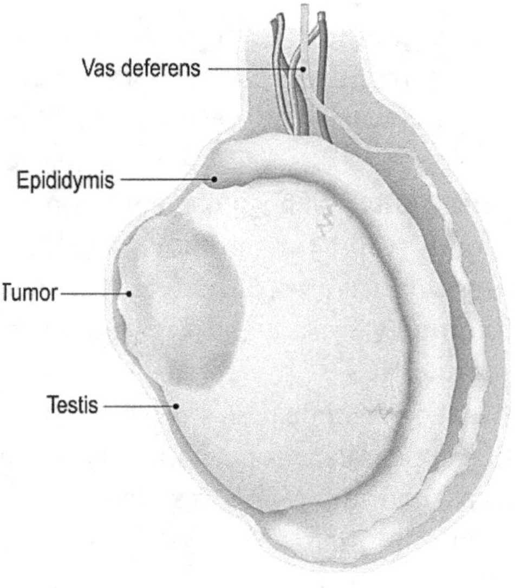

There are few types of non-seminomas: choricarcinoma, embryonal carcinoma, teratoma and yolk sac tumors.

There are also rare testicular cancers that do not form in the germ cells.

Leyding cells that produce testosterone sertoli cell tumors arise from the sertoli cells that support normal sperm growth.

Types of testicular cancer: There are 3 types of testicular cancer include:

1- **Seminoma:** Seminomas tend to grow and spread more slowly than nonseminomatous germ cell tumors, although some Seminomas can grow rapidly.

Subtypes of semino include:

- **Classic seminoma:** 95 percent of Seminomas are classic
- **Spermatacytic seminoma:** Tend to occur in older men and has an excellent prognosis.

2- **Nonseminomatous germ cell tumors:** There are 4 main types of NSGCT that can appear alone, but most often appear as a "mixed" NSGCT:

- **Embryonal carcinoma:** Present in about 40 percent of tumors and among most rapidly growing and potentially aggressive tumor types. Embryonal can secrete HGC or alfafetoprotein (AFP).
- **Yolk Sac Carcinoma:** The most common type of tumor in children: responds well to chemotherapy in children and adults. Yolk Sac tumors almost always secrete AFP.
- **Choriocarcinoma:** Vary rare and very aggressive form of testis cancer, can secrete HCG.
- **Teratoma:** Most often appear as a mixed NSGCT, usually grow locality but can appear in retroperitoneal lymph nodes. Teratoma is chemotherapy and radiation - resistant and best treated with surgical removal.

3- Stromal tumors: Tumor can also develop from the supportive tissues around the germ cells in the testicle. These tumors are more, making up less than 5 percent of testis cancers, and have an excellent progosis if surgically respected. There are two types of stromal tumors:

- **Leyding cell tumors:** leyding cell tumors make the male hormone testosterone and are more often cure with the surgery
- **Sertoli cell tumors:** Sertoli cells support and nourish the developing sperm and are usually benign tumors.

Stages of testicular cancer:

- **Stage 1:** Stage 1 is the earliest stage of testicular cancer.
- **Stage 2:** In stage 2 the cancer cells have spread from the testicle into nearby lymph nodes in your tummy (abdomen) or pelvis.
- **Stage 3:** Stage 3 testicular cancer means that the cancer has spread to lymph nodes or other organs.

Causes of testicular cancer:

It is not clear what causes most testicular cancer.

Testicular cancer starts when something causes changes to the DNA of testicle cells. A cell's DNA holds the instructions that tell the cells what to do. The changes tell the cells to grow and multiply quickly. The cancer cells go and living when healthy cells would die as part of their natural life cycle. This causes a lot of extra cells in the testicle that can form a mass called tumor.

In time, the tumor can grow beyond the testicle. Some cells might break to other parts of the body. Testicular cancer most often spread to the lymph nodes, liver and lungs. When testicular cancer spread, it's called metastatic testicular cancer.

Nearly all testicular cancers being in germ cells. The germ cells in the testicle makes sperm. It's not clear what causes DNA changes in the germ cells.

Symptoms of testicular cancer: Signs and symptoms of testicular cancer include:

- Lump or swelling I either testicle
- A feeling of heaviness in the scrotum
- A dull ache in the lower belly or groin
- Sudden swelling in the scrotum.
- Pain or discomfort in a testicle or the scrotum
- Enlargement or tenderness of the breast tissue
- Back pain.

How is testicular cancer treated: treatment for testicular cancer depends on the type of testicular cancer and how far it has spread.

You will usually need the affected testicle surgically removed in an option called an Orchiectomy.

Aloboratory will then examine the tissue to confirm the type of cancer and check how advance it is.

After the surgery, you may not need any further treatment, apart from close monitoring. In some cases, you may need chemotherapy or radiotherapy to kill any cancer cells that may have spread to other parts of the body, you may also need further surgery.

Prevention of testicular cancer: Testicular cancer can't be prevented: Unlike some other cancers, there are currently no recommended screening exams for Testicular cancer. It is recommended you consult a self - exam in a warm shower once a month. If you notice changes in the testicles, seek medical attention.

CHAPTER 13
HEART CANCER

Primary heart tumors are abnormal growth in the heart. They are very rare.

According to the European Society of Cardiology (ESC), they are found in less than 1 out of 2000 autopsies.

Most tumors that form in the heart are not cancerous. Some heart tumors can be cncererous. Cancer that begins in the heart is most often sarcoma, a type of cancer that originate in the soft tissues of the body. Heart cancer (malignant primary cardiac tumor) is extremely rare.

Heart cancer results from a heart' tumor like angiosarcoma or another cancer that spreads to heart. This rare cancer causes heart failure, pericarditis and arrhythmias. Cancer can spread to the heart from the organs or through blood (leukemia).

Types of heart cancer

The different types of heart cancer that are prone to occur in the human body

- **Myxom:** It is usually a benign (noncancerous) heart tumor occurring on the upper part of the heart. Maximum primary heart tumors are maximas, commonly, these are seen in the women between 49 and 60 years of age and can be inherited through family.
- **Primary cardiac lymphoma:** A rare form of malignancy, primary cardiac lymphoma involves only the heart and pericardium without extra cardiac organs. Abnormalities such as a trial arrhythmias and AV blocks are common in this disease.

The treatment normally follows multiagent anthracycline-based chemotherapy.

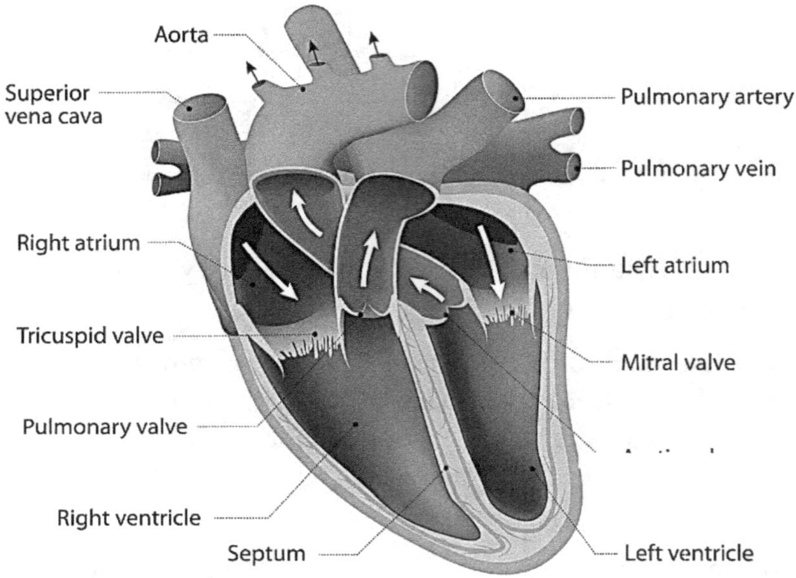

- **Pericardial Mesothelioma:** Another extreme form of the cancer, pericardial mesothelioma, occurs on the pericardium. It doesn't occur because of metastasis from other body parts. However, limited research shows risk generated from radiation exposure, virus 40 exposures etc.

- **Angiosarcoma:** A rare type of cancer, angiosarcoma usually forms in the lining of the blood and lymph vessels. Most commonly, it occurs in the right atrium, interfering in the functions of the neighbouring organs. It often results in pericardial effusion, heart failure and cardiac tamponade, surgical treatment can be the only way out of this.

Symptoms of heart cancer: The following list shows some common heart cancer symptoms, which one should not neglect at any cost.

- Fever and chills, fatigue, night sweating, Weight loss, and joint pain.
- Blood flow obstruction, causing fatigue, shortness of breath, chest pain and dizziness.
- Heart muscles dysfunction, causing Swollen legs, chest pain, and weakness and breathing shortage.
- Heart condition blockage, with slow or fast heartbeats, faint or fatigue, leading to the cardiac arrest.
- Embolus or blood clots traveling from heart to lungs, brain arm or legs.

Causes of heart cancer:

Scientists believe that certain people are more prone to this primary heart cancer because of their genes, but we are still learning about the genetic basis of most of these cancers. The cause may be related to mutation in a gene called protection of telomerase protein 1 (POT 1).

- **Angiosarcoma:** A rare type of malignant (cancerous) soft tissue tumor. The cause of angiosarcoma is unknown, although radiation and some toxins may play a role.

Stages of heart cancer:

- **Stage 0:** Means there is no cancer, only abnormal cells with potential to become cancer
- **Stage 1:** Means the cancer is small and only in one area
- **Stage 2 and 3:** Means the cancer is larger and has grown into nearby tissues or lymph nodes
- **Stage 4:** Means the cancer has spread to other parts of your body.

Treatment options for heart cancer: When possible, surgical removal is the treatment of choice for all the primary heart tumors

Benign tumors:

Most of these can be cured if the tumor be completely removed.

- When tumor very large or these are multiple tumors, removing part of it that isn't inside the heart walls can improve or eliminate symptoms instead of surgery

- Some types can be followed yearly echocardiograms instead of sury if they are not causing symptoms

Malignant tumors:

- Because they grow rapidly and invade important heart structures, they can be very difficult to treat.
- Unfortunately, most are not found until surgical removal is no longer possible.

Secondary heart cancer:

- By the time heart metastases are found, the cancer has usually spread to other organs too and isn't curable.
- Metastatic disease in the heart cannot be removed surgically.
- Palliative care with chemotherapy and radiation therapy is frequently the only option.
- If a pericardial effusion develops, it can be removed by placing a needle or small drain into the fluid collection.

Prevention of heart cancer: How diet can affect health and cancer risk.

Nutrition matters, both the terms of heart health and cancer risk. Here are some tips on how to modify your eating habits to protect your heart, prevent cancer and promoter overall wellness

- **Adopt a plant-** based diet. Eat plenty of fruits, vegetables, beans, outstand whole grains
- Limit your consumption of processed meats. Even very lean cuts of sodium, which can cause your blood pressure to sky- rocket. Additionally, the preservatives and compounds that form when meat is smoked or cure can be increased the risk of developing stomach and colorectal cancer.
- **Avoid empty calories:** consuming foods and beverages that are low in the nutrients and high in sugar can lead to both, weight gain and nutritional deficiencies. In particular drinking sodas and other sweetened beverages can easily lead to an excessive consumption of sugar, which can increase heart disease and cancer risk factors above and beyond.

CHAPTER 14
BREAST CANCER

Breasts cancer occurs when breast cells develop mutations and begin to divide and multiply. People may first notice a lump in the breast, discoloration, texture changes or other symptoms.

Breast cancer is one o the most common cancers that affects women and people assigned female at birth. It happens when cancerous cells in your breast multiply and became tumor. About 80 percent breast cancer cases are invasive, meaning a tumor may spread from your breast to other areas of the body.

Breast cancer typically affects women age 50 and older but it can also affect women and people AFAB who are younger than 50. Men and people assigned male at birth (AMAB) may also develop breast cancer.

Substantial support for breast cancer awareness and research finding has helped create advances in the diagnosis and treatment of breast cancer. Breast cancer survival rates have increases, and number of deaths associated with the decrease is declining largely due to factors such as earlier detection, a new personalized approach to the treatment and better understanding of the disease.

A breast cancer is made up of 3 main parts: lobules, ducts, and connective tissue. The lobules are the glands that produce milk. The ducts are tubes that carry milk to the nipple. The connective tissue (which consists of fibrous and fatty tissue) together.

Breast cancer is a disease in which cells in the breast grow out of control. There are different kinds of breast cancer depends on which cells in the breast turn into cancer.

Most breast Cancer begin in the ducts or lobules. Breast cancer can spread outside the breast through blood vessels. When breast cancer spread to other parts of the body, it is said to have metastasized.

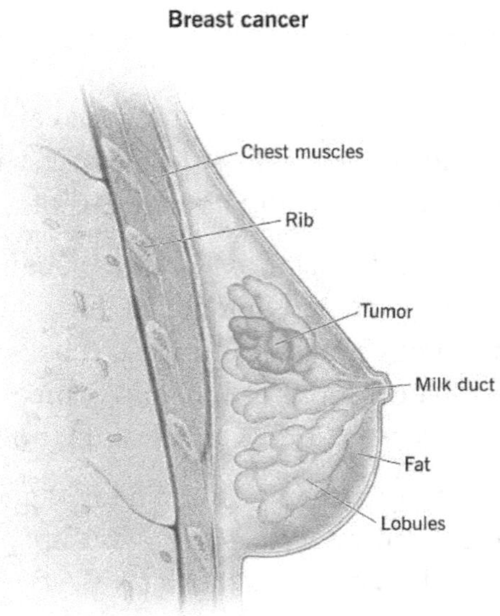

Scope of the problem:

In 2020, there were 2.3 million women diagnosed and 685000 deaths globally, there were 7.8 million women alive who were diagnosed with the breast cancer in the past 5 years, making it in the world's prevalent cancer, breast cancer occurs in every country of the world in women at any age after puberty but with increasing rates in later life.

Breast cancer mortality changed little from 1930s through to the 1970s when surgery alone was the primary made of treatment (radical mastectomy). Improvement in survival began in the 1990s when countries established breast cancer early detection programmed that were linked to comprehensive treatment programs including effective medical therapies.

Breast cancer in India:

How common has ranked among Indian females with age adjusted rate as high as 25.8 percent per 100000 women and mortality 12.7 per 100000 women. Data reports from various latest national cancer registries were compared for incidence, mortality rates with the latest study reports, India's highest cancer rate is listed in the state of Kerala. Other states with high cancer rates in India include Mizoram, Haryana, Delhi and Karnataka. Mizoram accounted for the highest cancer death rates.

In India, the incidence of breast Cancer has increased significantly. There was almost a 50 percent rise in the incidence between 1965 and 1985.

The estimated no of cases in India in 2016 was one lakh eighteen thousand.

The total no of living breast cancer cases in the same year was more than five lakhs twenty-five thousand. As per recent studies, tend to this disease is rising in younger women.

According to epidemiologic data, more than 25 in every one lakh women develop breast cancer. It is due to poor life style and Excessive body weight can be the two major risk factors for breast cancer post- menopause etc.

Types of breast Cancer:

There are many types of breast cancer and many different ways to describe them.

Ductal or lobular carcinoma:

Most breast cancers are carcinoma, which are tumors that start in the epithelial cells that line organs and tissues throughout the body when carcinoma form in the breast, they are usually a more specific type called adenocarcinoma, which starts in cells in the ducts (glands in the breast that make milk).

In situ vs invasive breast Cancers:

The type of breast Cancer (ductal carcinoma in situ or DC is) is a pre- cancer that starts in a milk duct and has not grown into the rest of the breast tissue. The term invasive breast cancer is used to describe any type of breast Cancer that has spread into the surrounding breast tissue.

Ductal carcinoma in situ.: Ductal carcinoma in situ that we call it intraductal carcinoma. It is a no invasive or pre- invasive breast cancer.

Invasive breast cancer: The most common types are invasive ductal carcinoma. It makes up about 70 to 80 percent of all breast cancer.

Special types of invasive breast cancer: Some invasive breast cancers have special features or developed in the different ways that influence their treatment and outlook. These cancers are less common but can be more serious than other types of breast Cancer.

Tripple - negative breast cancer:

Tripple negative breast cancer is an aggressive type of invasive breast cancer in which the cancer cells do not have estrogen or progesterone receptors and also do not make any or too much of the protein called HER2. It accounts for about 15 percent of all the breast cancers

Less common type of breast Cancer:

There are other types of breast Cancers that start to grow in other types of cells in the breast. These cancers are much less common, and sometimes need different types of treatment.

Paget disease of breast Cancer: It starts in the breast ducts and spreads to the skin of the nipple and then to the areola.

Angiosarcoma:

Sarcomas of the breast are rare making up less than 1 percent of all the breast cancers. Angiosarcoma starts in the cells that line blood vessels or lymph vessels. It can involve the breast tissue or skin of the breast. Some may be related to prior radiation therapy in that area.

Phyllodes tumor; Phyllodes tumors are breast tumors. They develop in the connective tissue (stroma) of the breast, in contrast to carcinomas, which develop in the duct or lobules. Most are benign, but there are others that are maglinant.

Stages of breast cancer:

Stage 0: Stage zero means that the cancer was caught in early stages. The cancer began in the milk glands or breast ducts and has remained confined to the place itself. It is common to hear your doctors throw around the term in situ at this stage, which means that the cancer remains in the original place where it began.

Stage 1: This is still starting level, but from stage one, the breast cancer said to be invasive. This means that the cancer cell has broken free from where they began and have started attacking other healthy tissue.

Stage 1A: This means that cancer has spread into the nearby fatty breast tissue. It also indicates that the tumor, though, is no bigger than a shelled peanut. In many cases, it is also possible there is no tumor present at this stage

Stage 1B: At this stage, there are some cancer cells present, but in a very small amount. These have been found in some of your lymph nodes.

Stage 2: Stage 2, The cancer has already grown or spread, or it could be bad.

Stage 2A: This stage refers to the breast tumor to still be small, and in some cases, there might be no tumor even by this stage, there might be also no cancer in the lymph nodes, or it is possible that the cancer has spread to a maximum of 3 lymph nodes.

Stage 2B: By this stage, the breast tumor is getting bigger - about the size of the walnut or even as big as a line. It might or might be present in the lymph nodes.

Stage 3; By stage 3 of the breast cancer, the cancer has not yet spread to any other organs or to the bones. However, it is considered to be an advanced stage and it is now considered more challenging.

Stage 3 A: Cancer has spread to or it has enlarged the lymph nodes that are located deep in the breast. In some cases, there can be no tumor present, but in others, there could be a large tumor already present in the breast

Stage 3 B: This stage means that the tumor has properly grown into the skin or chest wall around the breast. It might not have spread to the lymph nodes yet.

Stage 3 C: It is also considered to be at the third stage C if fewer lymph nodes located outside the breast have been impacted, but lymph nodes inside the breast are already cancerous. Or enlarged.

Stage 4: This stage is often referring red as metallic, which means that the cancer has spread beyond the part of the body where it is first originated.

Causes of breast Cancer:

Some factors that increase your risk of breast cancer include:

- Increasing age
- Family history
- Inheritance of mutations in the genes
- Exposure to female hormones Starting your period before age 12
- Previous breast cancer diagnosis
- Past history of certain noncancerous breast conditions
- Being overweight
- Not enough physical activity.

Symptoms of breast cancer:

- A change in the size, shape or contour of the breast
- A mass or lump, which may feel as small as a pea.
- Lump or thickening in or near your breast under arm that persists through your menstrual cycle

- A change in the look or feel of your skin on your breast or nipple. Your skin may look dimpled, puckered, scaly or inflamed. It may look red, purple or darker than other parts of your breast.
- marble - like hardened area under your skin.
- A blood stained or clear fluid discharge from your nipple.

Treatment of breast Cancer:

- **Surgery:** Surgery is the primary breast cancer treatment, but. healthcare providers may use other treatments. Breast cancer surgeries include:

- **Mastectomy:** This can be relatively minor or relatively major operation, depending on how large the tumor is and how much tissue needs removed.
- **Lumpectomy:** A Lumpectomy removes cancer cells and a small margin of healthy breast tissue.
- **Breast reconstruction:** Breast reconstruction can happen right after a mastectomy or much later. You may need multiple surgeries over several months

2- **Chemotherapy:** Chemotherapy for breast cancer is one of the ways that healthcare providers treat the condition. You may receive chemotherapy before and after your surgery.

3- **Radiation therapy:** People who have breast cancer surgery often receive Radiation therapy afterward to eliminate cancer cells that remain after surgery.

4 - **Immunotherapy:** Healthcare providers may use immunotherapy to treat high - risk early stage and metastatic triple - negative breast cancer.

5- **Hormone therapy:** Healthcare providers may combine hormone therapy with treatment such as, surgery, chemotherapy or radiotherapy.

6- **Targeted therapy:** healthcare providers sometimes use targeted therapy as the front line or initial treatment. They may also combine targeted therapy with other treatments.

Prevention:

1. Keep weight in check
2. Be physically active
3. Eat fresh vegetables and fruits
4. Do not smoke
5. Breast feed if possible
6. Avoid birth control pills
7. Avoid hormone therapy
8. Tamoxifen and Raloxifene for women at at high risk.

CHAPTER 15

BONE CANCER

Bone cancer occurs when a tumor or a typical mass of tissue in a bone. These are called bone sarcomas.

Bone cancer is when unused cells grow out of control in your bone. It destroys normal bone tissue. It may start in your bone or spread there from other parts of your body (called metastasis).

Bone cancer is rare. Most bone tumors are benign, which means they are not cancer and don't spread to other areas of your body. But may still weaken your bones and lead to broken your bones or other problems.

Primary bone cancer is a rare type of cancer that begins in the bones. Around 550 new cases are diagnosed each year in the UK.

Bone cancer develops in the skeleton system and destroys the tissue.

The two main types are primary and secondary bone cancer:

In primary bone cancer, cancer develops in the cells of the bone. Secondary bone cancer occurs when cancers that develop elsewhere spread, or metastasize to the bones.

According to the National Cancer Institute, primary bone cancer accounts for less than 1 percent of all the cancers. Secondary bone cancer is more common.

Bone cancer can spread to distant organs, such as lungs.

Our bones are made up of two basic types of cells: Osteoblasts, which create and maintain new bone, and osteoclasts, which dissolve old bone. Normally, bone cells know when to grow and when to stop growing. But sometimes, abnormal bone cells develop and grow at an uncontrolled rate, forming tumor.

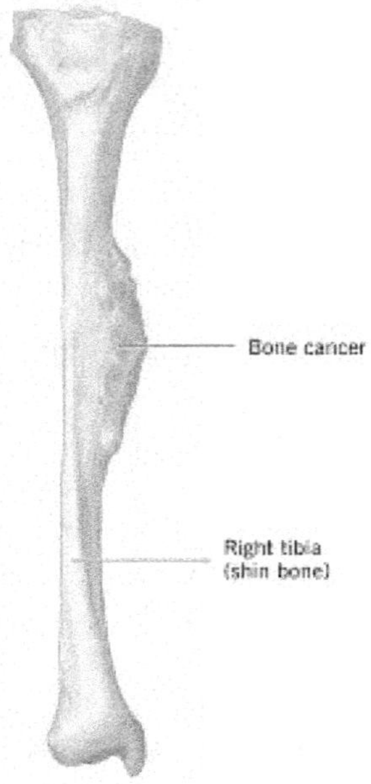

Stages of bone cancer: Bone cancer stages are based on 4 categories:

T (tumor): Describes the size of the original tumor.

N (Node): Indicates whether cancer is present in the lymph nodes.

M (Metastasis): Refers to the whether cancer has spread to other parts of the body.

Grades of bone cancer:

There are 4 grades designated for cancer.

Grade GX: The grade cannot be determined.

Grade 1 (G 1): Bone cancer closely resembles healthy tissue. This is considered a low - grade tumor.

Grade 2 (G 2): Bone cancer somewhat resembles healthy tissue. This is considered a high-grade tumor.

Grade 3 (G 3): Bone cancer look like very different from healthy tissue. This is considered high - grade tumor.

Types of bone cancer: Common types of bone cancers include:

Osteosarcoma: Generally, affects children and adolescents, but it can also occur in adults. It has a tendency to originate at the tips of the long bones in the arms and legs.

Osteosarcoma may also start in the hips, shoulders, or other locations. It affects hard tissue that provides the outer layer of the bones.

Osteosarcoma is the most common type of primary bone cancer, causing 2 in 3 bone cancer cases.

Ewing's sarcoma: This is the second common type primary bone cancer. It either begins in the soft tissues surrounding the bones or directly in the bones, and it often affects children and young adults.

The long bones of your body such as arms and legs- and pelvis are commonly affected.

Chondrosarcoma: Chondrosarcoma most commonly begins in the bones of the pelvis, thigh areas, and shoulder s of the older adults.

It forms in the subchondral tissue, which is the tough connective tissue between your bones.

These tumors are generally slow - growing. This is the last primary cancer involving the bones.

Multiple myeloma: This is the most common type of cancer affecting the bones. However, it's not considered a primary bone cancer because it begins in the plasma cells. It occurs when cancer cells grow in the bone - marrow and cause tumors in various bones. Multiple myeloma usually affects older adults

Causes of bone cancer:

The exact reason why this happens often not known, but certain things can increase your chance of developing bone cancer, including: previous radiotherapy treatment, other bone conditions, such as Paget's disease of the bone, rare genetic conditions, such as Li - Fraumeni syndrome.

Bone cancer symptoms: Signs and symptoms of bone cancer include:

- Bone pain
- Swelling and tenderness near the affected area
- Weakened bone, leading to fracture.
- Fatigue

Treatment of bone cancer:

Some bone cancers are treated with just surgery; some with Surgery and chemotherapy, and radiation therapy.

Surgery: In the most cases, this involves special techniques to remove the tumor in one single piece, along with small portion of the healthy tissue that surrounds it the surgeon replaces the lost bone with some bone from another area of your body, with material from bone bank or with a replacement made of metal and hard plastic.

Bone cancers that are very large or located in a complicated point on the bone may require surgery to remove all or part of the limb (amputation). As other treatments have been developed, amputation is becoming less common. If amputation is needed, you will likely to be fitted with an artificial limb and go through training to learn to do every day task using your new limb.

Chemotherapy:

Chemotherapy uses strong anti - cancer drugs, usually delivered through a vein (intravenously), to kill cancer cells. However, this type of treatment works better for some forms of the bone cancer than for others.

For example, chemotherapy is generally not very effective for chondrosarcoma and Ewing's sarcoma.

Radiation therapy:

Radiation therapy used high - powered beams of energy as X - ray, to kill cancer cells, during radiation therapy you lie on the table while a special machine moves around you and aims the energy beams at precise points on your body.

Radiation therapy is often used before an operation because it can shrink the tumor and make it easier to remove. This, in turn, can help reduce the likelihood the amputation will be necessary.

Radiation therapy may also be used in people with bone cancer that cannot be removed with surgery, after surgery, radiation therapy may be used to kill any cancer cells that may be left behind.

For example, with advanced bone cancer, radiation therapy may help control signs and symptoms, such as pain.

Prevention of bone cancer.

Bone sarcoma prevention while it is always good to maintain a healthy weight and quit smoking or using Tabacco, currently. Exercise may play a role for prevention of bone sarcoma.

CHAPTER 16

COLON CANCER

Colon cancer develops when tumors growth form in the large intestine. It often produces no symptoms in the early stages.

A cancer o colon or rectum, located at the digestive tract is lower end. Early cases can begin as non - cancerous polyps. These often have no symptoms but can be detected by screening. For this reason, doctors recommend screening for those at high risk or over the age of 50 or even earlier if a family history of colon is present.

Colon cancer develops from certain polyps or growth in the inner lining of your colon. Healthcare providers have screening tests that detect pre - cancerous polyps before they can become cancerous timers. Colon cancer that's not detected or treated may spread to other areas of your body. Thanks to screening tests, early treatment and new kinds of treatment, fewer people are dying from colon cancer.

Your colon wall is made up of layers of mucous membrane, tissue and muscle. Colon cancer starts in your mucosa, the inner most lining of your colon. It consists of cells that make and release mucus and other fluids. If these cells mutate or change, they may create a colon polyp

Over time, colon polyp may become cancerous (it is usually taking about 10 years to form a colon polyp). Left undetected and/ or untreated, the cancer works its way through a layer of tissue, muscle and the outer layer of your colon may also spread to other parts of your body lymph nodes or your blood vessels.

Colon cancer is the third most common cancer diagnosed in the U.S. According to the U.S centers assigned male at birth (AMAB)

are slightly more likely to develop colon cancer than women and people assigned female at birth (AFAB).

Colon cancer affects more people who are members of other ethnic groups or races.

Colon cancer typically affects people age 50 and older. Over the past 15 years, however, the number of people age 20 to 49 with colon cancer has increased by about 1.5 percent each year. Medical researchers are not sure why this is happening.

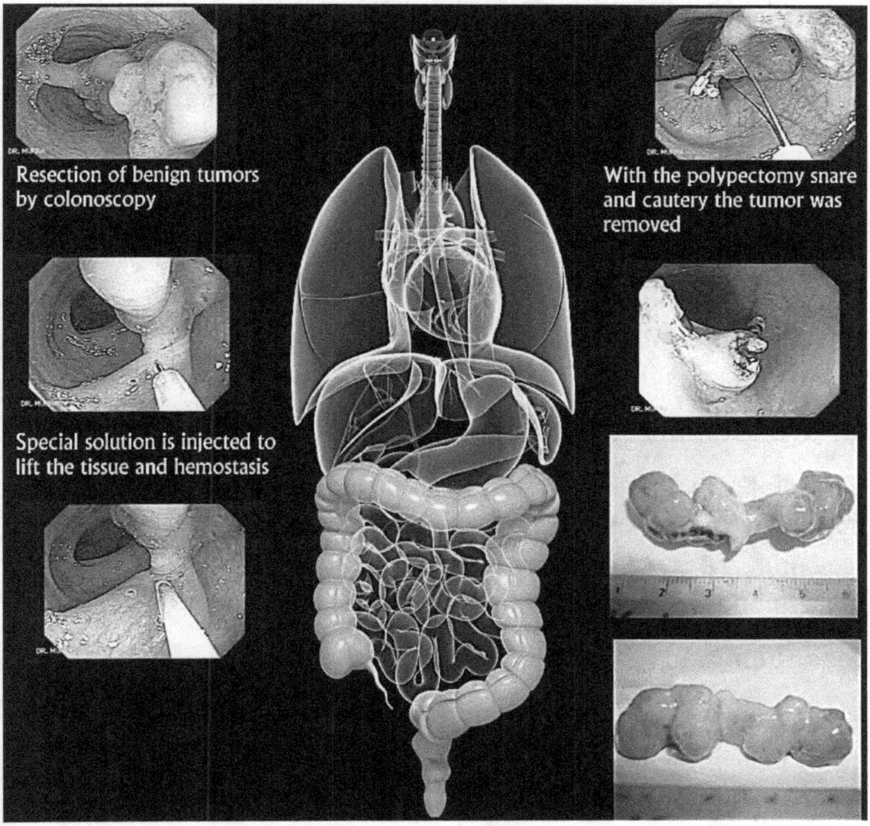

Stages of colon cancer: The stages develop as follows:

Stage 0: Also known as carcinoma in situ, at this point, the cancer is in a very early stage. It has not grown further than the inner layer of the colon and will usually be easy to treat.

Stage 1: Cancer has grown into the next layer of tissue.

Stage 2: cancer has reached the outer layer of the colon but has not spread beyond the colon.

Stage 3: Cancer has grown through the outer layer of the colon and reached 1 to 3 lymph nodes. It has not spread to distant sites.

Stage 4: Cancer has reached other tissues beyond the wall of the colon. As stage 4 progresses, colon cancer reaches distant parts of the body.

Types of colon cancer Adenocarcinoma:

The vast majority of colon cancer is adeno carcinoma. This is a cancer of cells that line the inside surface of the colon.

Carcinoid tumors: Carcinoid tumors start in the hormones producing cells in the intestines.

Gastrointestinal stromal tumors:

Gastrointestinal Stromal tumors can be a type of soft tissue sarcoma that can be found anywhere in the gastrointestinal tract but is rare in the colon. These tumors can be also other types of sarcoma that start in the blood vessels or connective tissue of the colon.

Lymphoma:

Lymphoma is a cancer of the immune system. It more commonly starts in the lymph nodes but can start in the colon.

Heredity colon cancer:

About 5 to 10 Percent of people get colorectal cancer because of specific mutations in the genes that are passed from parents to children, which are referred to as heredity.

Mask's colon cancer experts may offer you genetic testing to see if you have hereditary mutations in your genes that can increase your cancer risk. Whether you should have this testing is based on an assessment of your personal risk.

Causes of colon cancer:

Usually, cells follow an orderly process of growth, division, and death. Cancer can develop when cells grow and divide uncontrollably and do not die at the normal point in their life cycle.

According to American Cancer society, researchers are unsure the exact cause of the colon cancer, but certain factors may increase the risk.

Cancer happens as a result of changes in DNA within cells. Certain genes called oncogenes help cells stay alive, grow, and divide. Tumor suppressor genes help regulate cell division and cell death.

Changes to DNA can affect oncogenes and tumor suppressor genes, resulting in the multiple gene changes that may lead to colon cancer.

Polyps are growths that form on the inside of the colon. The polyps are noncancerous, but cancer can begin with some types of polyps.

If a person has type of noncancerous polyp, they have an increased risk of developing colon cancer. These polyps form on the inner walls of the large intestine.

Cancerous cell may spread from the malignant tumors to other parts of the body through the blood and lymph systems.

These cancer cells can grow and invade healthy tissue nearby and throughout the body in a process called metastasis. The result is more serious, less treatable condition.

Factors may increase the risk of colon cancer:

- Older age
- Black race
- A personal history of colorectal cancer or polyps
- Inflammatory bowel diseases

- Inherited syndromes that increase colon cancer risk
- Family history of the colon cancer
- Low fiber, high fat diet No exercising regularly.

Symptoms of colon cancer:

Many people with colon cancer do not have symptoms at first. When symptoms appear, they will like depend on the cancer's size and where it is in the large intestine.

Symptoms of colon cancer can include:

- A change in the bowel habits, such as more frequent diarrhea or constipation.
- Rectal bleeding or blood in the stool
- Ongoing discomfort in the belly area, such as cramps, gas or pain.
- Feeling that the bowel doesn't empty all the way during bowel movement.
- Weakness or Tiredness.
- Losing weight without trying.

Treatment of colon cancer:

The treatment for colon cancer includes:

Endoscopic treatment:

Often, polyps are safely removed during a colonoscopy. Some very large polyps may be removed without surgery by specially trained gastroenterologists known as therapeutic Endoscopists. If polyps were large, your doctor may have marked the polypectomy (polyp removal) Site with the special Inka during the colonoscopy. Marking the area can help during subsequent surveillance colonoscopies.

For patients with large polyps or more than three polyps, follow up colonoscopies should be performed more frequently. Consult your doctor your recommended screening schedule

Surgery:

The treatment of choice for colon cancer is surgical resection, which involves removing the cancer through surgery. Surgery is performed to remove the cancer completely and reconstruct the bowel, if possible, so your post operative bowel function is normal or near normal.

If the cancer is completely removed during surgery and confined to be early-stage disease, no further treatment is needed. If cancer cells are found in the surrounding tissue or lymph nodes, your doctor may recommend adjuvant chemotherapy.

Chemotherapy:

Chemotherapy drugs travel through the bloodstream to destroy tumor cells that may have broken away from original tumor and could begin to grow again elsewhere in the body.

They may be administered orally or intravenously.

Chemotherapy can be used at various stages of colon cancer treatment, so, sometimes, chemotherapy is given prior surgery to shrink a tumor and reduce the extent of surgery.

In more advanced cancers, you may need a course of chemotherapy following your surgery. This type of chemotherapy is generally ad mistered on an outpatient basis.

Chemotherapy may also be used after surgery. For more patients, chemotherapy can make radiation more effective in the treatment of colon cancer (Radiotherapy is not commonly used for colon cancer treatment)

Prevention of colon cancer:

- Take control
- Get screened. Getting regular screening tests for colon cancer is the single best way to protect yourself from the disease.
- Physically active
- Do not smoke
- Maintain healthy weight
- Avoid alcohol
- limit red meat especially process meat

CHAPTER 17

BLADDER CANCER

Bladder cancer is a common type of cancer that begins in the cells of the bladder. The bladder is a hollow muscular organ in the lower abdomen that stores urine.

Bladder cancer is a relatively rare form of cancer that starts in the lining of your bladder. There are many ways to treat bladder cancer, including surgery that removes bladder cancer. Bladder may come back after treatment, so people with bladder cancer

should be vigilant about following up with their Healthcare providers. Healthcare providers can treat early - stage bladder cancer - cancer that's found and treated before it can spread but about 75 percent of early -stage bladder come back.

Bladder cancer is the fourth common cancer affecting men and people designated male at birth (DMAB). Men and people DMAB are four times more likely to develop bladder cancer than women and people designated female at birth DMAB who do have bladder cancer typically have advanced forms of disease because they do not know about the bladder cancer symptoms.

According to the bladder cancer advocacy network, women are less likely to pay attention to the blood in their pee (hematuria), the first and most important bladder cancer symptoms, because they associated blood in pee with common gerontological issues.

Bladder cancer typically affects people age 55 and older. On average, people are 73 when they are diagnosed with bladder cancer. Men and people DMAB who are white are two times more likely to develop bladder cancer than men and people DMAB who are black.

STAGES OF BLADDER CANCER

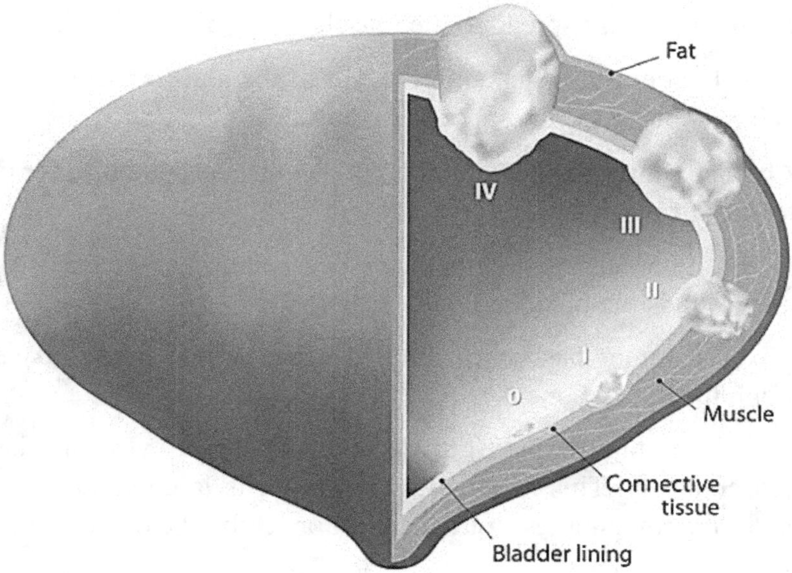

Stages of bladder cancer.

TX: primary tumor cannot be evaluated

T 0 (T zero): There is no evidence of primary tumor in bladder

T a: This refers to non-invasive papillary carcinoma. This type of growth often is found on the small section of tissue that easily can be removed with TURBT.

T is: This stage is carcinoma in situ (cis) or " flat tumor" this means that the cancer is only found on or near the surface of the bladder. The doctor may also call it non - muscle - invasive bladder cancer, superficial bladder cancer, or non-invasive flat carcinoma. This type of bladder cancer often comes back after treatment, usually as another non-invasive cancer in the bladder.

T 1: The tumor has spread to the connective tissue (called the lamina propria) that separates the lining of the bladder from the muscles beneath, but it doesn't involve the bladder wall muscle.

T 2: The tumor has spread to the muscle of the bladder wall.

T 2 a: The tumor has spread to the half of the muscle bladder wall, which may be called the superficial muscle

T 2 b: The tumor has spread to the deep muscle of the bladder (the outer half of the muscle)

T 3: The tumor has grown into the peri vesical tissue (the fatty tissue that surrounds the bladder)

T3 a: The tumor has grown into the peri vesical tissue, as seen through the microscope.

T3 b: The tumor has grown into the peri vesical tissue microscopically. This means that the tumor is large enough to be seen during imaging tests or to be seen or felt by the doctor.

T 4: The tumor has spread to any of the following abdominal wall, the pelvic wall, the prostate or seminal vesicle.

T 4a: The tumor has spread to the prostate, seminal vesicles, uterus or vagina. Surgical removal of the tumor may still be possible in this stage.

T 4b: The tumor has spread to the pelvic wall or the abdominal wall. Surgical removal of the tumor may not be possible in this stage.

Types of bladder cancer:

The bladder cancer is categorized by a number of types, depending on where exactly it forms, along with other factors. The most common type bladder cancer is transitional cell (urothelial) carcinoma (TCC). This type accounts for about 95 percent of bladder cancer. The cancer cells of this type look like the urithelial cell lining the inside of the bladder.

Subtypes of the most common type of bladder cancer.

There are two types of TCC outlined below.

Papillary carcinoma: grows out from the inner surface of the bladder toward the hollow center in the finger - like. Projections, often, these tumors are called non-invasive papillary cancers, they don't grow into the deeper layers of the bladder wall. When papillary TCC is very low grade, it may be called papillary neoplasma of the low malignant potential, and these bladder cancers treatments typically have positive outcomes.

Flat carcinoma: This type of TCC doesn't grow out of the urothelial toward the center of the bladder. Rather, flat carcinomas remain of the surface of the bladder wall. If a flat carcinoma is confined to the urothelium, it is called non-invasive carcinoma or flat carcinoma in situ.

Carcinoma in situ: Refers to a group of abnormal cells that have not spread from the location where they first formed, although they may later spread into normal tissue and become cancer in situ, also in situ cancer or cancer in situ, is different from invasive carcinoma, which has spread to surrounding tissue. It also differs from metastatic carcinoma, whis has spread throughout the body to the other tissues and organs. In general, carcinoma in situ is the earliest form of cancer, and is considered stage 0.

Causes of bladder cancer:

Some factors that can increase your risk of bladder cancer include:

- Smoking tobacco
- Older age
- Being male
- Work place exposure to certain chemicals called amines, benzene products. These are used in dying in the textile, petrochemical and rubber industries etc.
- use of chemotherapy drugs cyclophosphamide
- previous radiotherapy to the pelvic area.
- Diabetes treatment using the drug pioglitazone.
- Family history
- Chronic urinary tract infection.

Symptoms of bladder cancer:

The most common symptoms of bladder cancer is blood in the urine, which usually occurs suddenly and is generally not painful.

- Problems emptying the bladder
- Need of pass urine often
- Lower Abdominal or back pain.

Treatment of bladder cancer:

Staging: Staging describes the extent of cancer in your body.

Most common staging system used for bladder cancer is the TNM system which describes the stage of cancer from 1 to 4 stage. Determining the stage of your cancer helps your doctors plan to best treatment for you.

Types of treatment:

Superficial bladder cancers are treated with the surgery and / or immunotherapy or sometimes chemotherapy.

Surgery: (transurthral resection) is done using a cystoscope which has a wire loop which the doctor uses to remove any tumors. Other ways to kill the cancer cells can include burning the base of the tumor or high energy laser to damage or Kil the cells.

Immunotherapy:

Non-invasive bladder cancers can also be treated with immunotherapy. A vaccine called Bacillus Calmetter - Guerin, developed to prevent tuberculosis, can be used to stimulate your immune system in order to stop or delay bladder cancer.

Chemotherapy:

Drugs are used to destroy or damage cancer cells, chemotherapy drugs are instilled into the bladder cancers, chemotherapy drugs are instilled into the bladder (intravesical chemotherapy) Invasive bladder cancers are most commonly treated with surgery, although radiation therapy is an alternative treatment. In some cases, chemotherapy may be added.

If surgery is not in option, the cancer may be treated with or without alone (platinum and gem citable).

Palliative care:

In some cases of bladder cancer, your medical team may talk to you about palliative care.

Palliative care aims to improve your quality of life by alleviating systems of cancer with trying to cure the disease.

As well as showing the spread of bladder cancer, palliative treatment can relieve pain and help manage systems. Treatment may include radiotherapy or other drug therapies.

Prevention of bladder cancer:

- Smoking cessation, that's number one stop smoking or if you are exposed to second hand smoke, reduce that as well

There is some evidence that dietary proteins high in fruits and vegetables such as Mediterranean diet, may help reduce the risk of bladder cancer.

There is evidence that drinking a lot of fluid - mainly water - might lower the risk of bladder cancer.

CHAPTER 18

KIDNEY CANCER

Kidney cancer is a cancer that begins in the kidneys. Kidneys are two bean - shaped organs, each about size of the first.

Every person has 2 kidneys, which are located above waist on both sides of the spine.

These radish - brown, bean - shaped organs are each about the size of a small fast. They located closer to the back of the body than to the front.

The kidney filter blood to remove impurities, excess minerals and salts, and extra water.

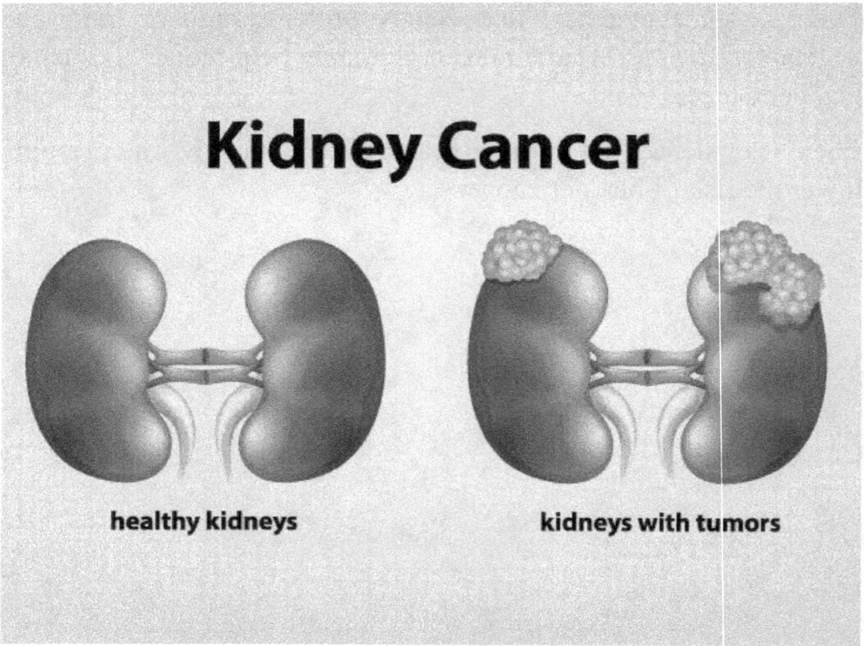

Every day, the kidney filter about 200 quarts of the blood to generate 2 quarts of urine. The kidneys also produce hormones that help control blood pressure, red blood cell production, and other bodily functions.

Kidney cancer begins when healthy cells in one or both kidneys change a mass called a renal cortical tumor. A tumor can be malignant tumor, indolent, or benign. A malignant tumor is also cancerous, but this type of tumor rarely spreads other parts of the body.

A benign tumor means the tumor can grow but will not spread.

Stages of the kidney cancer:

There are 4 stages of kidney cancer T 1 to T 4:

T 0: Means there is no evidence of primary tumor in the kidi.

T 1: is divided into T a and T 2b

T 2: is divided into T2a and T2

T 3: is divided into T 3a and T 3 c

T 4: means the cancer has spread further than the tissues around the kidney. NX means lymph nodes cannot be assessed.

Types of kidney cancer:

Renal Cell carcinoma (RCC) is the most common type of kidney cancer, accounting for approximately 85 percent of the malignant kidney tumors. In RCC, cancerous (Malignant) cells develop in the lining of the kidney tubules and grow into a mass called tumor. Like many other cancers, the growth begins small and grows larger over time. RCC typically grows as a single mass, where a kidney may contain more than one tumor, or tumors are fond in both kidneys at the same time.

Subtypes of Renal cell carcinoma (RCC). There are over a dozen subtypes of Renal Cell carcinoma that are identified by examining the tumor under microscope. The most common types are:

- **Clear cell -** approximately 75 percent of individual cells appear very pale or clear under the microscope.
- **Papillary -** approximately 10 Percent to 15 percent of people have live this form: These cancers form little finger like projections (called Papillae).

These are two types of papillary tumors.

- **Chromophobe -** approximately 5 percent cases. These cells are larger and have prominent cell borders and can appear pink or clear.
- **Clear cell papillary -** approximately 2 to 4 percent all cases. A new subtype with features of the both papillary and clear subtypes. These are often less aggressive.
- **Collecting duct**- approximately 1 percent of all cases. Aggressive type arising from the collecting system that forms regular tubules.
- **Medullary -** approximately 1 percent cases. Very aggressive type often occurring in young African American with sickle trait.
- **Unclassified -** approximately 2 to 3 percent of tumors that do not fit into any other categories.

Other types of cancerous kidney tumors (non renal cell):

Renal cell carcinoma makes up 95 percent of kidney tumors. Less common types of cancerous tumors in the kidney include:

- Urithelial carcinoma, arise from the renal pelvis and resemble bladder cancer cells. These are genetically similar to urothelian cancer of the bladder and have similar risk factors such as cigarette smoking and occupational exposures and certain causing chemicals.
- Wilm tumor, a rare pediatric malignancy in children 2 to 5.
- Renal sarcoma, a rare type of kidney cancer less than 1 percent arising from the connective tissue.
- Benign (non-cancerous) kidney tumors

Causes of Kidney cancer:

The causes of kidney cancer not known, but factors that put some people at higher risk are:

- Smoking- smokers have almost take the risk of developing kidney cancer as non- smokers.
- Work place exposure to chemicals such as arsenic and some other metals.
- A family history of the kidney cancer.
- Being overweight or obese.
- High Blood Pressure
- Having advanced kidney disease
- Be a being male- men are more likely to develop kidney cancer

Symptoms of kidney cancer:

In many cases, people may have no early symptoms of kidney cancer. As the tumor grows the larger, symptoms may appear. You may have one or more of these kidney cancer symptoms.

- Blood in your urine
- A lump in your side or abdomen
- Loss of appetite
- A pain in your side that doesn't go away
- Weight loss that occurs for no reason
- Fever that lasts for weeks isn't caused by cold or other infection
- Extreme fatigue.
- Anemia
- Swelling in your ankles or legs
- Shortness of breath
- coughing up blood
- Bone pain.

Treatment of kidney cancer:

Kidney cancer treatment options vary depending on the severity of cancer present.

Most often cancer is treated through surgery where the doctor eradicates the tumor from the body.

The surgery done could be simple or moderate, depending on the size and location of the tumor. Some of the treatment options for kidney cancer are-

- **Radical Nephrectomy -** It is a surgery performed to remove the infected kidney entirety along with the healthy tissues and lymph nodes surrounding it. This procedure conducted by an incision or through laparoscopy, which involves the insertion of thin tubes with camera attached to it.
- **Conservative Nephrectomy -** During the surgery the doctor targets to remove any the infected part of the kidney along with the small portion of the healthy tissues and lymph nodes. The remaining part of the healthy kidney is left behind to heal itself this process is known as Nephron sparing nephrectomy.
- **Non - surgical treatment -** kidney cancer can be cured without surgery non- surgical treatment methods are-

Cryoablation - this process is done by freezing that cancer - causing cell with the help of liquid nitrogen. This process is carried out by injecting special needles into the kidney tumor with the help of ultrasound scan images. The liquid nitrogen is passed through the hollow needle to feez the infected cells, which destroy them eventually.

Radiofrequency ablation - During this process, a particular probe is passed through the skin to reach the kidney tumor with the help of ultrasound images. Once the probe is placed in the targeted location, an electric current passed through the probe and then into the tumor cells to burn them.

Immunotherapy - The body loses the capability to fight against the cancer cells blind the immune system cells present in the body. This process can be reserved with the help of drugs like interferon and Aldesleukin, which are synthetic version of chemicals present in the body.

Targeted therapy - Targeted therapy helps in blocking particular unusual signals present in the kidney cancer cells and prevents them from multiplying.

Some of the drugs involved in targeted therapy are sorafenib (Nexavar), bevacizumab (Avastin), Axitinib (Inglyta), Pazopanin (Votrient), Sunitinib (Sutent), and Cabazontinib (Cabometyx). These play a vital role in blocking blood vessels that help in treating the cancerous cells. The other drugs such as Temsiolimus (Torisel) and Everolimus (Afjnitor) are target to block signals that help in the multiplication of cancer cells.

Radiation therapy - Radiation therapy is usually used to kill cancer cells that have spread to other parts of the body such as nearby organs, bones and brain. This therapy is done with the help of high powdered X- ray beams which brings the symptoms of kidney cancer under control. All treatments have their own set of side effects. Before undergoing these, it is recommended to clear all the doubts the treatment with the receive oncologists.

Prevention of kidney cancer:

- stop smoking
- Maintain healthy weight
- Control high Blood Pressure.
- Limit work place exposure to chemicals.

CHAPTER 19

SKIN CANCER

The abnormal growth of skin cells. Most often develops on skin exposed to sun. But this form of cancer can also occur on areas of your skin not ordinarily exposed to the sunlight.

Skin cancer happens when something changes how skin cells grow, like exposure to ultraviolet light. Symptoms include new bumps or patches on your skin, or changes in the size, shape or color of the skin growths. Most skin cancer is treatable it caught early. Skin cancer is a disease that involves the growth of abnormal cells in your skin tissues.

Normally, as skin cells grow old and die, new cells form to replace them, when this process doesn't work as it should - like after exposure to ultraviolet light from the sun - cells grow more quickly.

These cells may be noncancerous (benign), which do not spread or cause harm, or they may be cancerous.

Skin cancer can spread to nearby tissue or areas in your body if it is not caught early. Fortunately, if skin cancer is identified and treated in early stages, most are cured. So, it's important to talk with your healthcare provider if you think you have any signs of skin cancer.

The skin is the body's largest organ, skin has several layers are the epidermis (upper or outer layer) and dermis (lower or inner layer). Skin cancer begins in the epidermis.

Melanoma of skin is the 17th most common cancer worldwide. It is the 13th most common cancer in men and the 15th most common cancer in women.

There were more than 150000 new cases of Melanoma of skin in 2020.

Non - Melanoma skin cancer is often underdiagnosed, and commonly treated within primary care and therefore likely to be under - reported in National Cancer Registry data.

The ten countries with the highest rates of both types of skin cancer in 2020.

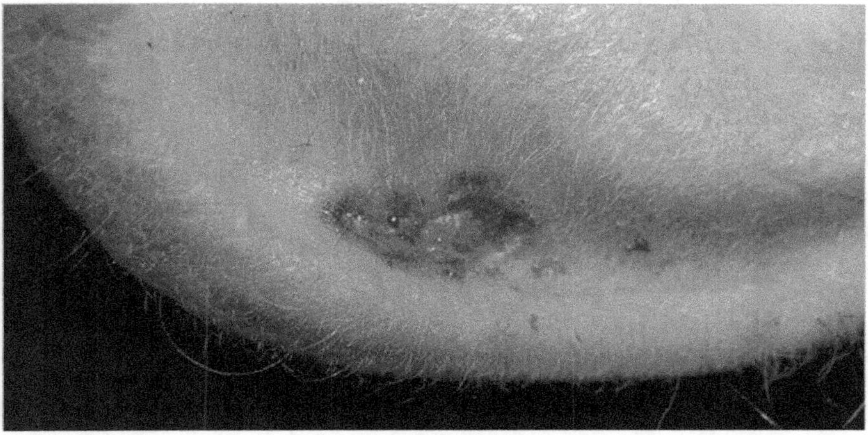

ASR equal to Age standardized rates.

These are the summary measure of the rate of disease that a population would have if it had a standard age structure.

Standardization is necessary when comparing populations that differ with respect of age has a powerful influence on the risk of dying from cancer.

Stages of cancer:

Squamous cell and basal cell skin cancers are staged as follow:

Stage 0: The cancerous cells are only present in the upper layer of the skin (Epidermis) and have not spread deeper into skin.

Stage 1: Tumor is 2 cm or less, has not spread to nearby lymph nodes and has one or fewer high-risk features.

Stage 2: The tumor is 2 to 4 cm, has not spread to nearby lymph nodes or the tumor is any size and has 2 or more high risk features.

Stage 3: The tumor is more than 4 cm or it has spread to one of the following.

- Subcutaneous tissue, which is the deepest, innermost layer of the skin that includes.
- Bone, where it has caused minor damage.
- a nearby lymph nodes.

Stage 4: The tumor can be any size and has spread to:

- one or more lymph nodes, which are larger than 3 cm
- Bone or bone marrow
- other organs in the body

Types of skin cancer:

The type of skin cancer a person gets is determined by where the cancer begins. If the cancer begins in the skin cell called basal cells, the person has basal cell skin cancer. When cells that give our skin, its color become cancerous, Melanoma develops.

1. Basal cell carcinoma (BCC):

This is the most common type of skin cancer:

- BCC frequently develops in people who have fair skin of color also get this skin cancer.
- BCC often looks like a fleshed colored round growth, pearl like bump, or pinkish patch of skin.
- BCCs usually develop after years of frequent sun exposure or indoor tanning.

BCCs are common on the head, neck, and arms, they can form anywhere on the body, including the chest, abdomen, and legs.

- Early diagnosis and treatment for BCC are important. BCC can grow deep. Allowed to grow, it can penetrate the nerves and bones, causing damage and disfigurement.

2. Squamous cell carcinoma (SCC) of the skin:

This is the second most common type of skin cancer.

- People who have light skin are most likely to develop SCC. This skin cancer also develops in people who have darker skin.
- SCC often looks like a red firm bump, scaly patch, or sore that heals and then reopens.
- SCC tends to form on skin that gets frequent sun exposure, such as rim of the ear, face, neck, arms, chest, and back.
- SCC can grow deep into the skin, causing damage and disfigurement.
- Early diagnosis and treatment can prevent SCC from growing deep and spreading to other areas of the body.

3- Melanoma:

Melanoma is after called " the most serious skin cancer" because it has tendency to spread.

- Melanoma can develop within a mole that you already have on your skin or appear suddenly as a dark spot on the skin that looks different from the rest.
- Early diagnosis and treatments are crucial.
- Knowing the ABCDE warning signs of Melanoma can help you find an early Melanoma.

Causes of skin cancer:

Most cases of skin cancer result from overexposure to ultraviolet light, including sun light and tanning beds, with the risk growing with the amount of exposure.

Besides ultraviolet light exposure, common skin cancer risk factors include:

- Weakened immune system, from viruses, diseases or immune - suppression therapy associated with organ transplantation.

Moles:

- personal or family history of skin cancer.
- Inherited conditions, such as xeroderma pigmentation.
- Smoking tobacco
- chemical exposure
- Basal cell nervous syndrome, also called Gorlin Syndrome
- Human Papilloma Virus (HPV)
- Kaposi sarcoma associated with herpesvirus
- Radiation therapy exposure
- Psoriasis treatment.

Symptoms of skin cancer:

Individuals should pay attention for warning signs of skin cancer, including:

- An unusual skin growth or sore that does not go away, such as nodule, rash or irregular patch on the surface of the skin.
- A pale patch of skin or a waxy or pearly white translucent bump on the head or neck, or a brownish scar or flesh colored lesion on the chest, which may be signs of basal cell carcinoma.
- Firm, rough lumps on the surface of the skin, sometimes developing more like a radish, scaly patch if nodule does not form, which may be signs of squamous cell carcinoma s.
- Red - or flesh-colored moles that are raised and grow quickly, which may be a signs of Merkel cell carcinomas.

Treatment of skin cancer:

Treatment depends on the staged of cancer. Sometimes, a biopsy alone can remove all the cancer tissue if it is small and limited to the surface of your skin. Other common skin cancer treatments, used alone on in the combination, include:

- **Cryotherapy:** your dermatologist uses liquid nitrogen to freez skin cancer. The dead cells Slough off after treatment.
- **Excisional surgery:** Your dermatologist removes the tumor and some surrounding healthy skin to be sure all the cancer is gone.

- **Moh's surgery:** Dermatologist removes only disease tissue, saving as much surrounding normal tissue as possible. Providers use this to treat basal cell and squamous cell cancers and, sometimes, other skin cancers that develop near sensitive or cosmetically important areas, like your eyelids, ears, lips, forehead, scalp, fingers or genital areas
- Curettage and electrodesiccation, your dermatologist uses an instrument with a sharp, looped edge to remove cancer cells as it scrapes across the tumor, then, they use an electric needle to destroy any remaining cancer cells. Providers often use this to treat basal cell and squamous cell cancers and precancerous skin tumors.
- **Chemotherapy:** your dermatologist or oncologist uses medications to kill cancer cells. Anticancer medications can be applied directly on the skin (typical chemotherapy) if limited to your skin's top layer of provided through pills or an IV if cancer has spread to other parts of the body.
- **Immunotherapy:** Your oncologist gives you medications to train your immune system to kill the cancer cells.
- **Radiation therapy:** Your radiation oncologist uses radiation (strong beams of energy) to kill cancer cells or keep them from growing and dividing.
- **Photodynamic therapy:** Your dermatologist coats your skin with medications, which they activate a blue or red fluorescent light. This therapy destroys precancerous cells while leaving normal cells alone.

Prevention of skin cancer:

Ways to protect yourself from skin cancer include:

- Use a broad- spectrum sunscreen with a skin protection factors (SPF) of 30 or higher. Broad- spectrum sunscreen and protect against both UV - B and UV - A rays. Apply the sunscreen30 minutes before you go outside. Wear sunscreen every day, even a cloudy day and during the winter months.

- Wear hats with wide brims to protect your face and ears.
- Wear long - sleeved shirts and pants to protect arms and legs. Look for clothing with an ultraviolet protection factor label for extra protection.
- Wear sunglasses to protect your eyes. Look for glasses that look both UV - B and UV - A rays.
- Use lip balm with sunscreen.
- Avoid the sun 10 AM to 4 PM.
- Avoid tanning beds.
- Ask your healthcare providers or pharmacist if anyone of the medications.

Regular check all your skin for any changes in size, shape, or color of the skin growth or development of new skin spots.

CHAPTER 20

CERVICAL CANCER

Cervical cancer is a cancer that starts in the cells of the cervix. The cervix is the lower narrow end of the uterus to the vagina (both cannal) The cervical cancer usually develops slowly over time. Before cancer appears in the cervix, the cell of the cervix goes through the changes known as dysplasia, in which the abnormal cells begin to appear in the cervical tissue.

About 14000 people in United States are diagnosed with cervical cancer each year. People between the ages of 35 and 44 are most frequently diagnosed with cervical cancer.

The average age at diagnosis is 50. Around 4000 people die of cervical cancer per year.

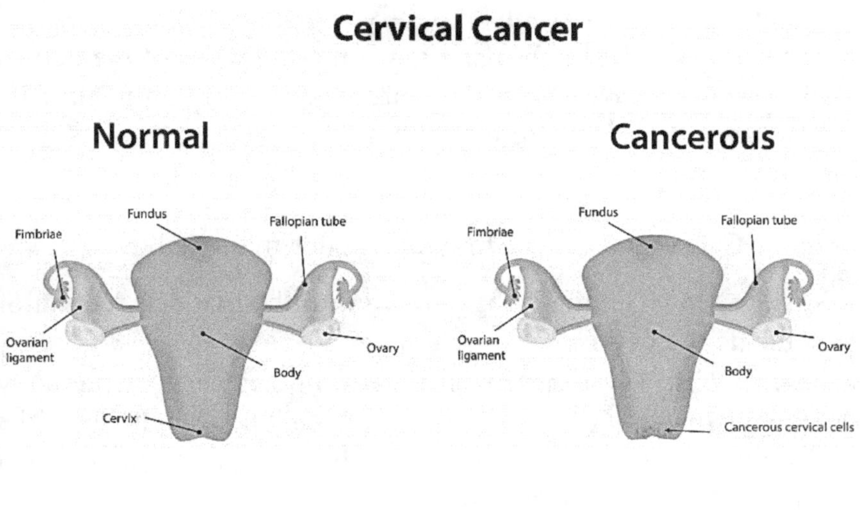

This rate is on the decline due to screenings and the HPV vaccine.

Stages of cervical cancer:

- **Stage 1 A:** The Tumor is in the cervix and can only be seen with a microscope. The tumor is not more than 7 mm wide.
- **Stage 1 A 1:** The tumor is not more than 3 mm deep and not more than 7 mm wide
- **Stage 1A 2:** The tumor is more than 3 mm, but not more than 5 mm deep and not more than 7 mm wide.

Stage 1 B: The tumor is in the cervix and can be seen without microscope but is bigger than a stage 1 A Tumor.

Stage 1 B 1: The tumor is less than 4 cm at its widest part.

- **Sage 1 B 2:** The tumor is more than 4 cm at its widest part

Stage 2 A: The tumor has grown outside the cervix and the uterus but has not grown into the walls of the pelvis.

- **Stage 2 B:** The tumor has grown outside the cervix and uterus into tissue next to the cervix and uterus. Tumor has not grown into the wall of the pelvis or lower part of the vagina.
- - **Stage 3 A:** Tumor has grown into the lower part of the vagina but not the walls of pelvis.
- **Stage 3 B:** The tumor has grown into the walls of the pelvis, blocks a ureter causing an enlarged kidney (hydronephrosis) or stops the kidney from working.

Or

Cancer has spread to lymph nodes in the pelvis.

- **Stage 4 A:** The tumor has grown into the bladder, rectum or outside the pelvis.
- **Stage 4 B:** The cancer has spread to other parts of the body (called distant metastasis), such as lymph nodes outside of the pelvis or to the lungs, liver or bone. This is also called metastatic cervical cancer.

Types of cervical cancer:

Cervical cancer is divided into two main types: Squamous cell carcinoma and adenocarcinoma. Each distinguished by appearance of cells under a microscope.

Squamous cell carcinoma: begin in the thin, flat cells that line the bottom of the cervix. This type accounts for about 90 percent of cervical cancers, according to the American Cancer society (ACS).

Adenocarcinomas of the cervix in the grandular cells that line the upper portion of the cervix. Cervical adenocarcinomas make up most of the remaining cervical cancer cases.

Causes of cervical cancer:

Cervical cancer begins when healthy cells in cervix develop changes in their DNA. A cell's DNA contains the instruction that tell a cell what to do - the changes tell the cells to multiply quickly. The cells continue living when healthy cells would die as part of the natural life cycle. This causes too many cells. The cell might form a mass called a tumor.

The cell can invade and destroy healthy body tissue. Intime, the cell can break away and spread to other parts of the body.

Most cervical cancers are caused by HPV, HPV is a common virus that's passed through sexual contact. For most people, the virus never causes problems. It usually goes away its own.

For some, though, the virus can cause changes in the cells that may lead to cancer.

Symptoms of cervical cancer:

Early on, cervical cancer usually doesn't have symptoms, making it hard to detect. Symptoms usually begin after the cancer has spread.

When symptoms of early - stage cervical cancer do occur, they may include:

- Vaginal bleeding after sex.
- Vaginal bleeding after menopause.
- Vaginal bleeding between periods or periods that are heavier or longer than normal.
- Vaginal discharge that's watery and has a strong odor or that contains blood.
- Pelvic pain or pain during sex.

Symptoms of advanced cervical cancer (cancer has spread beyond the cervix to other parts of the body) may include the symptoms of early- stage cervical cancer and

- Difficult or painful bowel movements or bleeding from the rectum when having a bowel movement
- Difficult or painful urination or blood in the urine
- Dull backache
- Swelling of the legs
- pain in the abdomen
- Feeling tired.

Treatment of the cervical cancer:

If you have been diagnosed with cervical cancer, you might have surgery, chemotherapy with radiotherapy (chemoradiotherapy), chemotherapy, radiotherapy or a targeted cancer drug, and an immunotherapy drug, what treatment you will have will depend on several things.

Surgery for cervical cancer: Surgery is one of the main treatments for cervical cancer. Surgery might include remaining of the most of the cervix (radical trachelectomy) or the womb (radical historectomy). Some people might have a pelvic exenteration for advanced cancer.

Radiotherapy for cervical cancer: Radiotherapy uses high - energy X- rays to kill cervical cancer cells. External radiotherapy alongside chemotherapy (chemoradiotherapy) is one of the main treatments for cervical cancer. This may be followed by internal radiotherapy (brachytherapy)

Chemotherapy for cervical cancer: Chemotherapy uses anticancer drugs to destroy cancer cells. The drug circulates throughout the body in the bloodstream.

Targeted and immunotherapy drugs for cervical cancer: targeted cancer drugs work by targeting the differences in cancer cells that helps to grow and survive. Other drugs help the immune system to attack cancer. They are called immunotherapies.

Controlling systems of advanced cervical cancer:

The symptoms of advanced cervical cancer depend on where the cancer is in your body. The team looking after you will offer support and treatment to help.

- **Pregnancy and cervical cancer:** treatment for the cervical cancer during pregnancy depends on type of cervical cancer, its stage, how many weeks pregnant you are and what your wishes are.

Prevention of cervical cancer:

The most important things you can do to keep prevent cervical cancer or to get vaccinated against HPV, have regular screening tests, and go back to the doctor if your screening results are not normal.

Human Papillomavirus (HPV), Immunization Project. Govt Set to roll out vaccine derive to fight Cervical cancer. campaign to target girls in 9-14 years age group, in 3 Phases over 3 years. Because India accounts for about 1.25 lakh new cases and 75000 death each year. Cervical Cancer is the second most Commen cancer among the women in India after breast cancer. As Per the news Indian Express dated 12 Jan 2024.

www.ingramcontent.com/pod-product-compliance
Lightning Source LLC
Chambersburg PA
CBHW062110160726
48282CB00026B/741
* 9 7 8 9 3 8 9 5 4 0 9 7 0 *